MW00612096

TO
DYE
FOR

TO DYE FOR

HOW TOXIC FASHION IS MAKING US SICK—AND HOW WE CAN FIGHT BACK

ALDEN WICKER

G. P. PUTNAM'S SONS
NEW YORK

PUTNAM
— EST. 1838 —

G. P. Putnam's Sons
Publishers Since 1838
An imprint of Penguin Random House LLC
penguinrandomhouse.com

ISBN 9780593422618
Library of Congress Control Number: 2023935924

Printed in the United States of America
1st Printing

To my mom,
who has invested so much in my happiness and success.
This book exists because of you.

And to my husband,
a constant source of love and support.
I'm so fortunate to have you on my team.

CONTENTS

PART IV: WHERE IT COMES FROM

PART V: HOW YOU CAN PROTECT YOURSELF

AUTHOR'S NOTE

My intent with this book is to expose the hidden effects of the chemicals in our clothes. I aim to be as accurate as possible, raising the alarm based on emerging research—without stoking unreasonable fear. In my quest for answers, I sought out researchers and textile professionals who were willing to be candid with me about what they were seeing in the industry. (Not such an easy task, to find independent and knowledgeable people who could speak their minds.) I also solicited stories from regular women about their bodies' reactions to fashion via the newsletter of my website, EcoCult, and social media platforms. Their stories provide compelling anecdotal evidence, but they are not statistically representative of the American experience.

In many cases, to protect the privacy and careers of the regular women and flight attendants who talked to me, I used either first names only or pseudonyms. Where I've done so, I've noted in the text.

I am not a medical professional, and this book is not intended to offer medical advice. If you suspect after reading this book that the chemicals used on your clothes may be behind some of your health problems, please speak to your doctor before making any decisions regarding medication or treatment.

INTRODUCTION

One day in September 2021, I found myself driving through the streets of a newish suburb an hour outside Phoenix. I had borrowed my mom's car, and its chipper navigation led me down long rows of identical stucco houses on identical streets with almost-identical desert landscaping of sand, rocks, succulents, and cacti.

I wasn't surprised that my quest had led me there. I knew the person I wanted to talk to had once lived in northern California, but she had subsequently developed a severe chemical sensitivity and then lost a bruising legal battle. The desert was the perfect place to retreat to.

People who suffer from sensitivities to mold, fragrance, or man-made chemicals often move to the desert, where the shimmering, dry heat kills all but the hardiest living things and soothes the myriad health conditions of an aging population. In fact, my own mom had moved to Phoenix from the Northeast for several reasons, but one was that her Raynaud's, an autoimmune-related condition where her circulation painfully retreats from her hands and feet during cold weather, had become hard to bear.

Out here, someone who has been driven out of their work and home by an invisible disability like chemical sensitivity can more easily afford their own patch of land and build a life that is free from the smells—dryer vents, cooking smoke, air pollution, lawn pesticides—that come with being up close and personal with your neighbors in America's more crowded and fecund cities and towns.

I pulled up in front of a small one-story duplex, shifted the car into park, and took a deep breath. For the past six months, I had called, emailed, and even sent a letter to the woman who lived there but hadn't gotten a response. This was my last attempt to introduce myself, to hopefully prove to her that I had her best interests at heart, and to draw her story out. Finally, I screwed up the courage, got out of the car, walked up to the door, and rang the doorbell.

After a minute of silence, the door swung open. I peered through the white metal screen door, still closed and locked. In the dim foyer, I could make out an older woman, thin and slightly stooped, wearing a white tee and black cotton shorts.

I introduced myself. "Hi. My name is Alden Wicker. I'm a journalist from New York. I'm working on a book about toxic fashion. I've been trying to get in touch with you. I want to hear your story."

"I know who you are," she said softly. She paused, collecting her thoughts. "You know, I have suffered from what they sprayed on those uniforms. My life was ruined. My husband left me for a younger, prettier woman." Her raspy voice trembled, teetering on the edge of breaking down. "My liver is damaged, my heart is damaged. I'm dying. I can't talk about it. I just can't. I can't go back to that experience again."

"Please," I said, close to tears myself. The gravity of what I had undertaken was hitting me anew, adding to my resolve to get the story down on paper before it was too late. "I've talked to the partner of an attendant who passed away. I want to know the story firsthand. Is there anyone else who would talk to me?"

"I'm so sorry. I asked everyone for help. My colleagues won't support me. They can't talk about it, either. I have to go. To a doctor's appointment, ironically," she said with some bitterness. "God bless you. God bless you." And the door clicked shut.

I stood for a moment in the bright sunshine, dazed, before walking back to the car. I had wanted to talk to this particular woman because she was the first airline attendant to file a lawsuit seeking redress for being poisoned by her uniform. She was also one of the first people in the world to have an inkling about just how sick our clothing can make us. Few believed her at the time. Even now, just a handful of people can even start to wrap their minds around what happened to her.

Back in the car, I tried texting some other potential sources. If this woman wouldn't talk to me, I knew I could find another. She was one of hundreds of attendants from Alaska Airlines who fell ill in 2011 when they received their new uniforms. And she was one of thousands from at least three other major airline carriers who, over the next decade, developed rashes, breathing problems, thyroid disease, hair loss, extreme fatigue, and a whole host of debilitating health issues that, in some cases, ruined their lives.

And it was all from wearing toxic uniforms.

My phone rang fifteen minutes later as I descended onto the highway that cuts through the hills into Phoenix's smoggy valley. It was a rep from the airline attendants union. She said if I would be careful to protect their identities, she would let me talk to the attendants.

———

I first learned about this story in 2019, when a radio producer reached out to me to ask if I could comment on a lawsuit filed by Delta employees against Lands' End, the apparel brand that made their uniforms.

At the time, I had no idea that clothing could make people sick. As a sustainable fashion and lifestyle journalist, I've been writing about almost all aspects of eco-friendly fashion since before it was cool. I've also been a longtime proponent of buying nontoxic cleaning products, "clean" beauty products made with simple and natural ingredients, and (most importantly) pesticide-free, organic food—as well as organic cotton.

I've built my career on the shoulders of authors like Rachel Carson, who, in the 1960s, ignited the modern environmental movement with her nonfiction book *Silent Spring.* The villains of her book were the fantastically toxic pesticide DDT, the chemical companies that spread disinformation about its supposed safety, and the government officials who allowed it to be used indiscriminately on roadside weeds.

The book's message was bleak—we were facing the possible extinction of the bald eagle, and of many other birds and wildlife. But what came after was an inspiration. Thousands marched in the streets, demanding a green revolution on the first Earth Day in 1970. That same year the Environmental Protection Agency (EPA) was founded, and in 1980, the federal government started demanding corporations pay for the cleanup of toxic sites. Today our rivers and air are cleaner than they have been since the Industrial Revolution.

I learned all this in high school, alongside the bad news about climate change and biodiversity loss, inculcating in me a sense that some battles had been won, but the war for the planet's future continued.

In college, as I studied journalism and business, I gave myself an elective of consumer health. I read Michael Pollan's *Omnivore's Dilemma* and Eric Schlosser's *Fast Food Nation.* They opened my eyes to how my food choices were damaging my health as well as the health of the soil and of animals. This information changed my life for the better, repairing my relationship with food, which had been exploited by a lifetime of being yanked between McDonald's and diet advertisements. I decided that if it matters where our food comes from, it probably matters where we get our other consumer products from, too. Right after college in 2009, I started blogging about all things eco, including beauty, travel, and fashion—mainly just to satisfy my personal curiosity and share what I found with the world. If I could change a few minds along the way, so much the better.

I wasn't alone in reassessing what I put on and in my body. Organic food promising to be free of pesticide residues is the fastest-growing sector in the food market, with sales hitting $57.5 billion in 2021. Beauty has followed close behind, with millions of women overhauling their entire bathroom cabinets in the past decade, throwing out legacy drugstore and department-store brands, which have toxic ingredients like phthalates and parabens, and investing in an ever-growing variety of natural products, which promise safety from hundreds of known carcinogens and hormone disruptors.

Women believe—with good reason—that the US government is failing to protect them from substances that can lead to birth defects, painful female reproductive issues, autoimmune diseases, and cancer. Influencers and beauty start-ups capitalized on these fears, peddling a potent mix of misinformation and expensive solutions that require chemistry and toxicology degrees to parse. The millions of women who follow these people and trends are investing a huge amount of money and time into the mystery of their never-quite-there health. They try elimination diets and "clean eating," DIY their beauty products, and spend thousands on creams and supplements, hoping that *this* will be the thing to banish their fatigue and period pain.

But the tide of change has spilled over the walled gardens of the wealthy. Even the largest, most affordable drugstore brands are now reformulating their beauty and cleaning products to be safer. And you can find organic milk at conventional grocery stores, too.

Yet fashion, a $2.5 trillion global industry, has somehow completely evaded the same scrutiny.

It's not that we've been totally unaware of the nasty chemicals used to produce clothes. The heavy pesticide use on cotton crops—with farmers in India and the US getting cancer as a result—was always a hot topic in green circles. Everyone in the industry knows that workers in textile mills and leather tanneries have been known to develop skin lesions and breathing problems. In 2011 (the last time industrial pollution in China was measured and shared publicly), textile manufacturing was up there with the paper and chemical industries as the third-biggest industrial contributor to China's water pollution. The same year, Greenpeace launched a campaign to bring awareness to the toxic chemicals flowing out of the pipes of these factories, turning rivers across Asia the color of the season, with red, purple, and blue plumes. In 2012, Greenpeace followed that bombshell with a report that found nonylphenol ethoxylates (NPEs, toxic endocrine disruptors that have been phased out of detergents) in 89 out of the 141 clothing samples it bought and tested, plus phthalates and restricted azo dyes on others. Every brand, from Giorgio Armani to Calvin Klein and H&M, was guilty of selling toxic clothing.

Awareness of the chemicals used on and in clothing might have kept growing if not for another fashion scandal that engulfed the news cycle.

In 2013, the Rana Plaza garment factory in Bangladesh collapsed, killing more than eleven hundred people. As pictures of family members clutching the bodies of workers pinged around the globe, Western consumers realized that real people, not robots, are hunched over sewing machines making their clothes. The next year, nonprofit Fashion Revolution launched an international day to commemorate the deaths, and its #whomademyclothes campaign was seen by 275 million people in 2018 alone. In the following years, the plight of factory workers continued to dominate the headlines.

Ask many popular sustainability influencers and actresses today what their aha moment was about the human toll of fast fashion, and they'll cite the 2015 documentary *The True Cost*. This film exposed how garment workers labor overtime for poverty wages so that we can buy ultracheap clothes, only to throw them away after a few wears. It was a shocking revelation that changed hearts and minds—and consumer behavior.

My career as an investigative fashion journalist grew alongside this consumer movement. I was writing for ever-larger outlets, and my blog EcoCult's traffic and newsletter subscriber base was growing by leaps and bounds as both regular people and industry professionals searched for guidance. But I was starting to question whether we could really shop our way out of climate change and worker exploitation. Everything seemed to be headed in the wrong direction, even as #sustainablefashion became the hottest trend on Instagram.

By the time 2019 rolled around and I got that email about the uniforms that were making flight attendants sick, I was flummoxed. The general understanding was that when it came to chemicals, it was cotton farmers and garment workers who were affected, not the end user. It was a problem *over there*. That clothing could cause such serious and acute health problems for the relatively privileged people wearing the clothes was news to me. I called up a few smart people in the fashion industry who I thought would know more, but nobody was able to give me any information.

The internet didn't help, either. Sure, there were a few articles from wellness influencers and "integrative health coaches" with some scary claims, like there being enough pesticide residue on nonorganic cotton clothing to get you sick. I've never found any evidence of that. (But I have found evidence that a lot of certified organic cotton is fraudulent, sadly.) No reputable sources seemed to have spotted *this* story, of what can be put on the cotton—and, for that matter, polyester, nylon, wool, and viscose—many steps after it has been harvested and woven.

I declined to go on the radio show that day to discuss the issue—I'm not one to talk about things I don't know about—but my interest was piqued. What is in our clothing? Could there be a huge scandal hiding in plain sight, right on our shirtsleeves?

It appeared that no one else had cared to ask these questions, at least not publicly, anyway. But I've always taken the fashion industry—and the people affected by it—as a deadly serious topic. So I dug deeper. I learned that this lawsuit was just the latest of several against airlines and the makers of their new uniforms, going all the way back to Alaska Airlines and Twin Hill in 2012.

In early 2019, I convinced an editor at *Harper's Bazaar* to give me a story about toxic fashion, and during my reporting, I interviewed one particularly vocal attendant at American Airlines. Heather Poole is a bestselling author of a 2012 memoir, *Cruising Attitude: Tales of Crashpads, Crew Drama, and Crazy Passengers at 35,000 Feet.* She had started blogging and giving media interviews about her own downward health spiral, and in the process she had become a leader in a cross-airline movement for recognition of what was happening. She was making trouble—good trouble—for the four major airlines and three uniform brands that wanted to sweep the whole thing under the rug.

The American Airlines attendants got their uniforms at the same time in the fall of 2016. They wore it for several days in a row, slept in it on overnight flights, drove with it in their cars, hung it next to their beds in crash pads. And in the weeks and months that followed, many of them started getting sick. With so much time spent together in airplanes and on layovers, they could compare notes with their colleagues and recognize patterns. Heather created a Facebook group where they could share stories with attendants from other airlines. And yet, it still took quite some time for many of them to make the connection between their symptoms and the uniform.

But was this problem of "toxic fashion" isolated to the airline industry? Or were the attendants just the proverbial canaries in the coal mine, early detectors of a more widespread phenomenon?

I was trying to figure out whether the same thing could be happening to regular consumers, albeit on a less noticeable scale. It seemed so. If you were to buy one or more toxic pieces of fashion, you would probably never think to connect your headache or fatigue to your pretty new sundress or performance leggings. Connecting chronic illness like thyroid disease or a cancer diagnosis to a sweater? Impossible.

"You can't prove anything unless you have an extreme situation," Poole told me in 2019, as she sat at home on unpaid leave, pining to be back in the sky. "What's happening to me is probably happening to you. But you wouldn't even understand it or know what was causing it."

It occurred to me that, while beauty and cleaning products and packaged foods come with an ingredient list, fashion does not. Like many, I assumed that meant there wasn't much on or in clothing fabric that wasn't the fabric itself. Surely, if there was something to be worried about, the government would be on it. I mean, how complex could a pair of leggings or a T-shirt be?

Very complex, as it turns out. Fashion products have some of the most complicated and multilayered chemical profiles of any product you or I can buy—without a license, anyway. Multiple chemical substances are used to manufacture, process, weave, dye, finish, and assemble clothing and accessories. Each step in this daisy chain can leave a residue, either intentionally or unintentionally, on the item that you then sleep, sweat, and live in almost every hour of every day.

Even in the general population, there are clues that something isn't right. Consumers have reported chemical burns from tights and shoes to the Consumer Product Safety Commission (which rarely recalls anything as a result), and individuals have sued children's and lingerie brands for the same. People with diagnoses of multiple chemical sensitivity, mast cell activation syndrome, or dye allergies shop brands with good return policies, struggling to find clothing that doesn't make them break out in hives or rashes. We have an epidemic of autoimmune disorders, which can often start with a simple rash or mild asthma, before spreading and turning into devastating illnesses in which the immune system attacks the body, like Crohn's or psoriatic arthritis. We're covering our fashion with hormone-disrupting chemicals, and then wondering why couples are increasingly having to pay tens of thousands of dollars for medical interventions to get pregnant.

At least forty thousand chemicals are used commercially worldwide, yet only a small percentage of them have been checked for human and animal safety. Some researchers have warned that we are producing too many chemicals and at too high a volume, that we are "outside the safe operating space of the planetary boundaries" for man-made chemicals.

And the chemicals created from fossil fuels are also at least partly to blame for fashion's climate footprint. The chemical industry is now the largest industrial consumer of both oil and gas, and as we switch to electric cars and wind and solar energy, petrochemicals are predicted to drive half of all demand for oil by 2050.

These chemicals can be acutely toxic or hazardous, causing skin burns or asthma. But more often they do their dirty work over years of chronic yet infinitesimally small exposure. They can be carcinogenic (causing cancer), mutagenic (damaging your DNA and causing birth defects), or reprotoxic (causing reproductive issues). Sometimes your body can metabolize and pee out these chemicals, and once in the water or soil, they eventually break down and go away. But others accumulate in your body and in the environment, lasting for decades or, in the case of perfluorinated chemicals like the kind in stain-resistant finishes, forever. Some of them mimic hormones, causing a little-understood cascade of health effects ranging from unwanted weight fluctuations and fatigue to infertility and chronic disease.

What's worse is that they are an invisible menace, infiltrating our air, water, homes, and bodies. In fact, there's now a term for the invisible world of synthetic chemistry that lives inside us: *the human toxome.*

How could it be that we know so little about something that plays arguably the most intimate role of any consumer product in our daily lives? The textiles and materials that caress our most private body parts have become duplicitous: beautiful and alluring, yet dangerous. Only the faintest clues—a whiff of caustic odor here, a disconcertingly bright color there, a plasticky hand feel—hint at their true nature.

In the following pages, you'll meet more than a dozen people who have discovered—whether through their research or lived experience—what the chemical industry and in some cases the fashion industry have been trying to hide from us. They are flight attendants, researchers, fashion professionals, garment workers, doctors, partners, and mothers who are part of a small but growing international club of people who know, beyond a doubt, that the clothing we put on our bodies can be—and often is—toxic.

By the end of the book, I think you'll be in this club, too.

Most importantly, I hope this will serve as proof for Western consumers that there is no "over there." What happens in Bangladesh and Morocco and Guatemala has very real effects on us, too. We are all connected, via these things too tiny to see, and via an issue almost too huge to comprehend.

Maybe, with your help, we can start an inclusive movement for fashion—and for a planet—that is safe, nourishing, and free of toxic chemicals.

PART I

CANARIES IN THE COAL MINE

CHAPTER 1

IN CASE OF EMERGENCY

Chemicals in the Not-So-Friendly Skies

Mary stopped the beverage service cart in the aisle and nudged the brake on with her foot. Smiling, she leaned toward the passenger by the window and took in a breath before asking them if they would like anything to drink.

At that moment, she started to choke, and buried her face in the elbow of her navy-blue jacket as she continued to hack. Gathering herself, she apologized profusely, poured herself some water, and continued with some effort to serve drinks. After she managed to finish the service, she stood in the back galley, wondering what the heck was going on. Lately, she had been coughing all the time, even though she had no other symptoms of a cold or flu. It was the spring of 2011, almost a decade before the Covid pandemic started making its way around the world in airplane cabins.

Mary (not her real name, to protect her job) was otherwise healthy and active. She had a gym membership and liked to go hiking in the verdant mountains that rise thousands of feet above Seattle, where she lives and where Alaska Airlines, the company she works for, is headquartered. Well, she hiked when she had time. Mary had a hectic work schedule, flying six days a week all over the US. Sometimes she would work fourteen days in a row, which lasted anywhere from six to twelve hours, with just enough time for a quick dip in the hotel pool and a sleep during her layovers. But by and large, she loved her job. "I drank the Kool-Aid," she said later. "I thought I mattered. I thought I was part of the family."

Mary, along with her twenty-eight hundred colleagues, had received a box from Twin Hill containing her new Alaska Airlines uniform a few months before, in late December 2010. When she pulled out about a dozen plastic-wrapped pieces, she judged it a big improvement over the old frumpy, bulky wool uniform made by M&H, an American uniform maker. These new pieces had a modern cut and were made with a sleek, polyester-wool blend fabric. What she didn't know is that while pure wool is naturally flame retardant, the new uniform's flame retardancy was provided by a chemical finish—and the fabric came with many other performance-enhancing chemicals, such as stain-proofing provided by Teflon.

Mary had heard senior attendants complaining that the new uniforms were giving them a rash. "I thought, *these people are just mad because they don't like change*," she told me a decade later. She was having her own breathing problems, but said, "I had not put two and two together. No one had ever heard of being poisoned by clothes before."

One of those senior attendants who was complaining the most was John, an attendant with twenty-five years of experience who lived in Long Beach, California, near his base of LAX. Back in 1986, John was a fifth-degree, black belt tae kwon do instructor when a friend invited him along for an interview to be a flight attendant at a small airline. He'd gone just for fun, but when he was offered the job, he took it and never looked back. The very next year, the airline was bought and absorbed into Alaska Airlines. By his midfifties, John had softened a bit around the middle but still had a handsome, boyish charm, with a square jaw, dimpled chin, and short brown hair.

According to his partner, Marco, John was low-key, even reserved, on the ground. But when he donned his Alaska Airlines uniform, he took on a different persona: gregarious, silly, charming. If he noticed a colleague was feeling down, he would go out of his way to make them laugh. At fast-food restaurants, he would order kids' meals so he could give the toys to fussy children on flights. He celebrated his colleagues' birthdays and put on funny hats for holidays.

John was a hard worker, and loved his job. When Alaska's insufficient maintenance of an older plane led it to crash off the California coast in 2000, killing everyone on board, John went right back to work. "It's just like getting thrown off a horse—you need to get right back on, otherwise you won't do it again," he told Marco.

John and Marco had met during one of John's layovers in San Francisco. They made it official with a domestic partnership in 2007, before it was legal for two men to be married in the US. John kept his home near LAX but, as an attendant with seniority, would select as many layovers in San Francisco as possible so that he had to spend only a few days a week away from Marco, who lived in the Bay Area.

"He wanted to keep working as long as possible. He loved his job," Marco told me by phone in 2021. "That all changed in 2010, when they issued those uniforms."

On a cool December day, John pulled the new uniform pieces out of the box and started trying them on in front of the mirror. Within the next two days, his whole upper body flushed with a rash, and he had trouble breathing, according to complaints he submitted later to the flight attendant union. He wore the outfit to work in January, before Alaska communicated the official rollout date, and he landed in the emergency room with severely compromised breathing and blisters on his arms. He came away from that ER visit with a $4,900 bill and a diagnosis of bedbug bites. Few had heard of a piece of clothing being toxic before. Rashes? Sure. That can happen when the pH balance of fabric is off. But landing in the emergency room from a blazer? The doctors had nothing to offer.

In fact, this wasn't the first time something like this had happened. In 2009, Transportation Security Administration (TSA) employees—the people who work the security checkpoints in airports across the US—started telling the American Federation of Government Employees that their uniforms gave them rashes, light-headedness, red eyes, swollen and cracked lips, and runny or bloody noses.

A TSA representative downplayed the issue. Less than 1 percent of the fifty thousand TSA workers were complaining, after all. And the Nashville-based manufacturer of their uniforms, VF Solutions, had the uniforms tested and said all substances, including formaldehyde, were below "acceptable limits."

"It's not a new fabric," VF Solutions' vice president for safety told the *Washington Post*. Just a typical cotton-polyester blend. There was no reason for these reactions to kick up now. But TSA agents were offered the option of 100 percent cotton alternatives. We don't know if John, his doctors, or even anyone at Alaska Airlines had heard about the TSA uniforms—I heard about them from another attendant who had done hours and hours of research.

All Alaska Airlines flight attendants were required to report to work in their new uniforms by February 23, 2011. Within days, Judith Anderson, an industrial hygienist in the Department of Safety, Health, and Security at the Association of Flight Attendants (AFA), started receiving emails and calls from members about the new uniforms and nasty reactions.

Anderson is slender and pale, with green eyes and straight, light-brown hair she keeps in a conservative sideswept crop. She has the air of a preschool teacher, with a soft voice that emanates both concern and gentle authority. Like the attendants she represented, Anderson tended to wear a conservative skirt suit and tights—with the addition of a perky scarf; you might find yourself asking her for soda water and pretzels.

In 1993, when Anderson graduated from college with a degree in chemistry and biopsychology, she started looking around for a master's program that would allow her to work in public health and have a real-world impact. When she learned about the field of industrial hygiene, it seemed like a great fit.

Anderson's second job out of school—after a stint in cancer research in British Columbia—was at George Washington University, helping the Center to Protect Workers' Rights assess chemical exposure of maintenance workers at a paper pulp mill. She remembers putting on steel-toed boots, walking inside a giant chemical digester, and seeing people welding without any respiratory equipment.

"It was appalling to see the conditions that some people work under," she told me by phone from her home office in Seattle in early 2022. She felt compelled to use her education and relative privilege to advocate for laborers.

So in 1999, when she saw a job posting at the Association of Flight Attendants—the largest flight attendant union in the world, representing tens of thousands of people from more than a dozen different airlines, including US Airways, Alaska Airlines, Hawaiian Airlines, and United Airlines—she was intrigued. But Anderson was also unsure that it would offer the kind of challenge and advocacy work she was looking for. "I thought, *How dangerous could this job be?*" she said. Sure, flight attendants work hard, and the struggles of working with the public in a stressful environment have been well documented, especially in recent years. But were their jobs and their working environments actually toxic in the literal sense? She wasn't so sure. "I had this glossy image of what it is to be a flight attendant," Anderson confessed to me.

But she quickly found out that flight attendants—and to a lesser extent, passengers—are often surrounded by a cocktail of toxic chemicals on the plane. And because they float above earth in workplaces not covered by the Occupational Safety and Health Administration, flight attendants actually need *more* advocacy from someone like Anderson, not less. She took the job and threw herself into the interesting, engaging work. It's a job she still holds today.

As an industrial hygienist working inside the airline industry, Anderson supports not just the airline employees but, in effect, the traveling public as well. For example, on cold days, the smell of de-icing fluid infiltrates the airplane cabin. Anderson has also worked on airborne illnesses, including SARS and COVID-19, and the simple danger of it being dangerously hot or cold in the airplane cabin.

And the AFA has been fighting since the 1970s to reduce the quantity and toxicity of pesticides that are sprayed up and down planes during stopovers to countries like Australia and India that have policies requiring it. In 1979, after some passengers experienced anaphylactic shock, the CDC stopped requiring routine disinfection on flights to Hawaii. In a small win in 2001, the AFA managed—with the help of the California Board of Health—to convince a large airline to stop spraying pesticides directly on the attendants' bunk beds in the large planes that do overnight flights to Australia. (Often the beds and passenger seats would still be wet when boarding started.)

But the "fume events" were what shocked and alarmed Anderson the most. That's when the jet engines start leaking hot oil into the air exchanges that run past the engines, and toxic fumes fill the cabin. Anderson receives weekly reports from crew members about "dirty sock smells" and smoke so thick it makes them cough, then develop headaches, brain fog, dizziness, and fainting.

Over the years, Anderson had developed close working relationships with the flight attendants from a dozen different airlines, from the young idealistic women working puddle-jumping commuter flights between small American cities to the seasoned attendants who serve champagne on jumbo jets to exotic destinations. If an attendant suspected they might have been poisoned on the job, Anderson was often the only sympathetic ear they could find.

Now, in 2011, pictures appeared in her inbox from Alaska attendants, of red patches of skin, swollen eyelids, and eyes crusted with pus. Unbeknownst to Anderson or the flight attendants, Alaska Airlines' customer service representatives were also having trouble with the uniforms. They filed a complaint with the Department of Labor & Industries in Washington State, where the airline is headquartered. The agency sent a letter to Alaska Airlines on March 3, describing the reactions.

In early March, John put on his uniform, and again, within minutes, he broke out in hives and couldn't breathe. It was clearly an ongoing problem. His manager encouraged him to see a worker's comp doctor, and he got one month of paid leave.

Alaska started demanding answers from Twin Hill, who had the uniforms tested and sent a memo to Alaska Airlines saying there were "no foreign chemicals" in the uniforms, meaning that everything that was on there had been put there on purpose. The oxford shirts contained formaldehyde at 24 parts per million (ppm), below the most stringent limit of 75 ppm, in Japan. They also had a Teflon coating, which made the uniforms stainproof. (That's the stuff on nonstick frying pans.)

By fall 2011, when several of Alaska's senior executives had a meeting with the AFA, the story had changed. Judith Anderson recalls them explaining that a few bolts of fabric had been contaminated during transit from Turkey to China with a chemical called TBP, or tributyl phosphate. She immediately recognized the name. Also known as phosphoric acid tributyl ester or tri-n-butyl phosphate, it's an ingredient in almost every hydraulic fluid used in the aerospace industry.

It also had shown up in fume events—something she was all too familiar with.

In work settings, TBP can cause skin problems; if inhaled, it can cause respiratory problems. It's also a potential endocrine disruptor, which means it could interfere with hormones and thyroid functioning. *What the heck is TBP doing in clothing?* Anderson wondered.

She started doing research and found out that, far from being accidental contamination, TBP is often used as a wetting agent and solvent in textile manufacturing. Greenpeace found it in a sample of polluted water issuing from a textile manufacturer into the Yangtze River delta during its explosive 2010 investigation into toxic runoff from apparel factories.

Alaska Airlines tried to assuage attendants' concerns by painting the TBP found in their uniforms as perfectly normal. It purchased uniforms by other brands and got them tested to show they also had TBP, albeit at much lower levels. And it offered $135 to all the flight attendants for dry cleaning. But experts told Anderson that dry cleaning wouldn't get rid of it. By July, Twin Hill's story had changed again. Now it was telling Alaska Airlines that the fabric had been contaminated in Turkey, and that the brand had severed its relationship with the Turkish fabric mill responsible. But these clothing reactions didn't seem to be isolated incidents—Anderson was getting emails from bank and hotel employees who were also having reactions to their own Twin Hill uniforms.

The thing was, Anderson couldn't find an official limit for TBP on textiles. Only Levi's specifies a limit for tributyl phosphate in garments: 50 ppm. The uniforms contained between 10 and 57 ppm, but Twin Hill didn't have to conform to another brand's voluntary and arbitrary standard. Instead, it hired a consulting company, Environ, which said the levels of TBP in the uniforms did not explain the symptoms that flight attendants were reporting.

So why were so many people getting sick?

Fashion's Dirty Secret

Judith Anderson was starting to discover the dirty secret of the fashion industry. In the United States, outside of California, there are vanishingly few legally enforceable standards that limit what kind of chemicals can be put on fabrics and then sold to adult consumers—or forced on employees. Instead, there are voluntary guidelines put together by private companies, industry groups, and a few multinational brands like Nike, Levi's, and H&M. And how do they determine what chemicals to look for and at what level they're safe for human health? Hard to say. Rarely are the limits based on robust research. More often they are the result of a few studies, sometimes on rats, sometimes on unfortunate employees at factories who are exposed to the chemical day in and day out. Sometimes, the limits are arbitrary best guesses or just industry "best practice."

That means someone at the fashion brands has guessed that the performance attributes of a chemical are worth any potential side effects to the wearer.

One day in May, Mary woke up with a rash spreading across her chest. She covered it with makeup and headed down to have breakfast in the hotel dining room with an older colleague.

"What's all this?" the senior attendant said, pointing to Mary's chest. Mary shrugged.

"You need to quit wearing the uniform, and you need to quit wearing it right now," the senior flight attendant said.

Mary protested, but the attendant fixed her with a stare usually reserved for an unruly passenger. "Take it from someone who's been here for a while and knows the route," Mary remembers him saying. "You're nobody. You're just a number. And you need to quit listening to what the company is telling you, get rid of that uniform, and go buy your own clothes." When Mary revealed that she had been coughing and getting migraines, the older attendant told her to get a notebook so she could start keeping track of her symptoms.

So Mary did. It took only a few weeks of notes to realize that her cough showed up only when she was at work, in her uniform. She went out and bought her own navy-blue suit pieces and white button-down shirts. At the time, her supervisor was sympathetic and helpful.

That would soon change.

That summer, John ended up in the ER again. Lesions that oozed blood crept up from his upper back to his collarbone, and then to his ears. His allergists and dermatologists didn't believe him when he said it was his shirt causing the problem. "We brought that uniform and said to the doctors, 'If you have an EpiPen, open the uniform and see what happens.' Every single one would just step back and say, 'We're not doing that, put this away.' Nobody even wanted to test the damn thing," Marco told me. John got a diagnosis of atopic dermatitis—a rash—and a prescription for steroid cream. When, in November 2011, John was taken off the plane because he couldn't breathe and was sent to the emergency room, Alaska Airlines denied that his condition was work related, according to Anderson and Marco.

"Literally overnight, you could tell that the legal team for the airline stepped in," Mary told me. "They sent out an email referencing anybody that had had a negative impact from the uniform as an 'individual sensitivity.' That was the new catchphrase. And then if you ever talked to a supervisor after that, [they would say,] 'Oh, I'm sorry you're having an *individual sensitivity*.' No, this isn't an individual sensitivity. I was poisoned."

By this point, Mary's eyes had become red and crusty. Despite this, she says her supervisors started pressuring her to put the official uniform back on.

Meanwhile, the AFA's Judith Anderson was trying to get help from the government, without much success. The Consumer Product Safety Commission said the flight attendants' workplace was regulated by the Federal Aviation Administration, not them, and forwarded the reports to the FAA, which passed them to the Occupational Safety and Health Administration, which told her to try the National Institute for Occupational Safety and Health (NIOSH), an agency that researches work-related injury and illness and makes recommendations on how to prevent them . . . but has no regulatory power. So in January 2012, Anderson asked NIOSH to look into the issue.

Even though Mary was no longer wearing the uniform, her troubles continued. With almost all her colleagues still wearing it, she struggled with migraine headaches, rashes, and eye issues. Bruises showed up in waves all over her body. She had trouble remembering basic words like *helicopter* or *doorknob*. Once, when she was visiting her parents, she stuttered so badly when she tried to ask them for the remote that she decided to make an appointment with a doctor for a cognitive test. It came back on the low end of the normal range.

"They blew me off," she said of the doctors she visited looking for answers. "They absolutely looked at me like I was a crazy person."

John also was reacting to something in the air. When he and Marco were waiting in a hotel lobby for a bus to the airport for a trip to Europe, John paused to speak to a couple of his colleagues who were wearing the uniform. He stayed several feet away from them, but by the time they got on the airport bus, John's throat was closing and Marco had to stab him with an EpiPen.

"A doctor has informed me if I wear those shirts again, knowing what they do to me, she will no longer provide treatment for this problem," John wrote in an email to Judith Anderson in early February 2012. "I don't believe she would do that. She just wanted me to understand the seriousness of the issue." He told Anderson he still had the offending shirt, and offered to send it to her. She gladly accepted, thinking that maybe his shirt could give her the answer.

"The action of having cut my shirt in half, packaging it, and labeling it this morning has caused a breathing reaction, swollen right eye, and rash with blood spots again on my left arm," he wrote to her.

Anderson had found out about a Washington State program typically used by employers to test workplace exposure to chemicals. She deconstructed some new, unworn Alaska uniforms—polyester lining and pockets, wool-blend jacket shells, cotton shirts and scarves—with ceramic scissors, which are sure to be free of toxic chemical contamination. Then she sent the sixty fabric samples to a lab at the University of Washington. The resulting report identified a total of ninety-seven chemical compounds in the uniforms—one fabric alone had forty-two different chemicals on it, including excessive levels of lead and arsenic in thirteen of the thirty-five fabric samples tested. The lab also found cobalt and antimony, restricted disperse dyes known to cause allergic reactions, the fossil-fuel chemical toluene at "low levels," and dimethyl fumarate, an antifungal that had recently been banned in the European Union. Plus, one blue sweater had hexavalent chromium, a carcinogenic heavy metal, on it.

The report said most of the substances were below typical levels that would cause irritation, but they could have had an "additive effect"—the concentration of dyes added together could exert a greater impact than each by itself—or a potential skin irritant like TBP could alter the skin's barrier and increase the chance of an allergic reaction.

This additive effect is something Anderson paid special attention to. She pointed out to me that the American Conference of Governmental Industrial Hygienists considers mixtures of chemicals when setting limits in the workplace. If all the chemicals in a particular mixture act on the same organ, or if they all cause the same health problems, then industrial hygienists consider their effects together.

But recommended chemical limits in the textile industry are set by considering most chemicals in isolation. If all of them are individually below recommended limits, then nothing, by their standards, is wrong—even if, combined, they exceed those limits. Conventional wisdom in the industry is that "the dose makes the poison." The trick is to find out what the safe limit is for each type of chemical and keep everything below that limit. By those guidelines—at least for the chemicals they had tested for—the uniforms were perfectly okay.

Anderson decided she needed the most respected lab in the field of textile toxicity—the Hohenstein Institute in Germany—to take a look at the uniforms. Hohenstein does testing for a nonprofit certification called Oeko-Tex, whose Standard 100 label establishes a standard of safety for consumers. And the limits it sets on how much of each chemical is safe to have on textiles has become a sort of official—if voluntary—guidance for the industry. The tests would cost the union thousands of dollars, but it would be worth it if it meant the uniforms would finally be recalled. Anderson packaged up uniform samples, including John's shirt, and sent them off to Germany.

When Anderson got the Hohenstein lab report in October 2012, she eagerly opened it and scanned the dense, jargon-filled document for an answer. It said that the dye Disperse Orange 37/76 was over the European Union's limit of 50 milligrams per kilogram by more than ten times. In fact, it was so high that it was outside the test's ability to measure it—the results listed it as "above 500 mg/kg." It's a known skin, respiratory, and eye irritant, so much so that the fashion industry had (supposedly) phased it out of use.

Anderson thought she might have her answer. But there was only one problem: the dye was present only in the pocket liner fabric. A toxic pocket didn't explain why attendants like Mary and John were getting rashes on their torsos, or why John was reacting specifically to the white button-down. And all the rest of the potentially toxic substances were under the lab's limits.

That same month, almost a year after it started its investigation, NIOSH finally gave Anderson its answer. After reviewing the records of seventy-eight attendants and the chemical analyses, it had failed to pinpoint the one chemical that could have caused all the dermatitis. It concluded that the percentage of attendants reporting skin problems did "not appear to be unusual" for an airline worker or even the general population. And anyway, they could have just noticed symptoms because of "heightened awareness," as NIOSH put it.

Anderson was incensed. "Affected flight attendants are not seeking an excuse to be sick or to not work," she wrote back. "NIOSH is comparing apples to oranges."

What she was saying is this: to conclude that the reactions were normal, NIOSH had compared the self-reported reactions from Alaska attendants (apples) to health surveys of Swedish attendants and general American workers (oranges). The general surveys would have asked a random sample of workers to check off all health effects that apply and so would have caught almost every little rash and episode of shortness of breath that workers had experienced during the preceding months. But it was clear that not all Alaska Airlines attendants who had a rash or shortness of breath while flying in the past year had reported it to the union. Only the attendants who were sick enough that it affected their life, who attributed their symptoms to the uniforms, and who felt confident they wouldn't be retaliated against by the airline, were filling out the forms. Furthermore, comparing flight attendants—who have a highly active job that requires them to push carts up and down the aisle and drag suitcases up and down airport staff stairs—to the general population—which includes those with disabilities and elderly people—is also not a fair comparison. It's a safe assumption that Alaska Airlines flight attendants were on average a pretty ablebodied bunch . . . until they weren't, suddenly and somehow all at the same time.

The thing is, Harvard researchers had collected the exact type of survey data Anderson would need from flight attendants at several airlines in 2007, including 684 Alaska Airlines attendants. Anderson contacted the researchers and asked them if they would do the next phase of their survey. If Harvard researchers could show that the incidence of symptoms jumped in Alaska attendants after they received the uniforms, that would be unassailable evidence that the uniforms were toxic. The researchers agreed, and they started sending out surveys.

"I knew, absolutely knew in my bones, that something was definitely wrong with these garments," Anderson said. "Alaska Airlines—and this is true of all the airlines since then—they wanted a smoking gun. They wanted one chemical to point to and say, *It's this. It's formaldehyde. And this explains everything.*" Anderson didn't have that. Instead, she had dozens of different chemicals, all with known or suspected different or overlapping human health effects, working in concert with each other.

Falling Down to Earth

The saga of the Alaska Airlines uniforms by Twin Hill was not an isolated incident.

The same thing happened when American Airlines introduced its Twin Hill uniforms in 2016. Then Delta and its Lands' End uniforms later that same year. Southwest and Cintas came next in 2017. (Alaska Airlines, American Airlines, and Southwest Airlines did not respond to my requests for comment.)

I spoke to sick attendants at every airline, and their stories were maddeningly familiar. They got rashes and asthma first, or dragging fatigue. They tried to play by the companies' rules. They got doctors' notes and approached their supervisors to ask to wear plain suits they bought with their own money instead. But according to the attendants I spoke to, the airlines only sometimes granted exceptions. For the anywhere from 8 to 22 percent of attendants who reported having adverse reactions, their best option was to work while sick, alongside their colleagues who continued to wear the uniforms. Draconian point systems based on missed workdays, regardless of whether they were due to the uniforms the airline was making them wear, forced attendants to choose between their jobs and their health. The airlines continually said that it was the fault of the attendants' own, too-sensitive bodies, and that there was no evidence the uniforms could make a typical person sick. The message was clear: get back on the plane, or find another job.

But what if it wasn't just an "individual sensitivity"? What if the chronic health problems they were experiencing were more common than anyone knew or wanted to admit, and were due to the very clothes on their backs?

The airline attendants are a near-perfect case study because they already operate in a controlled environment with few of the complex variables of an average person's life. Each airline switched all its attendants into new uniforms simultaneously, and each started receiving complaints not long after from a decent percentage of its attendants. The attendants wear the uniforms for up to twelve hours a day several days in a row and work on a set schedule inside near-identical workspaces with few external factors. In other words, they wear the same clothes, for the same amount of time, in the same location. During this time, they're in tight quarters with their own and their colleagues' uniforms for hours on end. It's as close as we're going to get to a control group—and their exposure levels are high enough, for some, to apparently cause acute and severe illness.

All these uniforms had a few things in common. They boasted water and stain repellency. They were anti-wrinkle, antifungal, and anti-odor and came in the bright, saturated colors of the airlines. In other words, they contained layer upon layer of nearly every newfangled chemical process on the market. And all those finishes and dyes seem to have made for a potent combination.

Or maybe it was the cheapness of these new uniforms? Or the

fact that they were all made in countries with lax chemical standards? The attorney representing Delta attendants, Bruce Max-
well, told me that Delta's Lands' End uniforms were made in
China, Malaysia, Sri Lanka, Indonesia, and Vietnam. Shipping
records show Twin Hill importing mainly from Sri Lanka, Indonesia, and Bangladesh, while Cintas has imported its polyester
dress shirts and sweaters from China and Vietnam.

To Judith Anderson, who was often on the phone with attendants from Delta and Southwest and giving informational webi-
nars, the answer was clear: as airlines negotiated the price of
uniforms down while demanding high performance, the brands
resorted to low-quality materials and manufacturers to preserve
their profit margins. "It never occurred to me in a million years
that you can get this sick from wearing clothes," Anderson told
me. Her quixotic journey to protect attendants from toxic fabrics
had led her to a frightening conclusion: no one is in charge of this
stuff.

Here's the thing—the uniforms are still just clothing. They're
made of the same fabrics, use the same dyes, and are made in the
same factories as regular mass-market clothing. You can also buy
wrinkle-free blouses at the mall and waterproof jackets at the outdoor store, and your fast-fashion jeans are likely treated with the
same fumigants to protect them on the trip from humid South
Asia to our shores.

"There are next to zero regulations for chemical content of
clothes in the United States," Anderson said. "I mean, there's a
handful of regulations in Europe on PFAS and flame retardants
and disperse dyes. But in the US, from what I can tell, it's very
much of a Wild West. Especially when you consider that almost all
clothing, fabric, manufacturing, and assembly takes place overseas,
it's surprising to me that there's just so little oversight."

The main difference between you and the flight attendants is
the variety of what's in your wardrobe. Instead of wearing the
same four or five uniform pieces as thousands of other people every

day, you cycle between dozens of different pieces a week. It's therefore harder to pinpoint the problem—to work out whether your T-shirt, underwear, or suit could be causing your tiredness, anxiety, or fertility issues. And even if you were wearing a toxic piece of clothing right now, how could you prove it was the cause of your mysterious health problems? There wouldn't be a clear before and after. You wouldn't have anyone to talk to and compare notes with. You wouldn't have an employer to complain to. You wouldn't have a union to test your outfit for you. You would be completely in the dark.

I wanted to see how widespread the acute health issues suffered by the attendants were in the general population. How many people were potentially getting sick from their wardrobes? Unfortunately, nobody has ever looked into this connection before. But the stats on the health of women (who do seem to be at higher risk) aren't good. In the US, one in eight women will develop breast cancer in her lifetime, and the same number will develop thyroid issues, characterized by fatigue, a slow or racing heartbeat, irregular periods, hair loss, forgetfulness, and weight gain or loss. (Until recently, when it was overtaken by colorectal cancer, thyroid cancer was also the fastest-increasing type of cancer in the United States.) About 70 to 90 percent of cancer cases are not genetic but attributed to environmental factors, including smoking, diet, and toxic chemical exposure.

Then there are the fertility issues: young women are struggling to have children more than ever, and while women are more likely to suffer from hormonal issues, men are also suffering from their own plummeting fertility crisis that threatens the survival of the human race. Researchers attribute these falling sperm counts to man-made chemicals in our environment. And many of those same chemicals are present in our clothes.

"We see the trends, but we cannot nail the trends to this and that chemical," Dr. Åke Bergman, a Swedish environmental toxicologist who specializes in endocrine disruptors, told me in early

2021. He was part of a task force convened in 2020 to advise Sweden on taxing toxic chemicals used in fashion. "There is an enormous use of a large number of chemicals. We strongly feel that there is a link between the exposures to these chemicals and the effects that are observed."

I asked Judith Anderson if she had ever had reactions to normal clothing before.

"Yeah, I mean, I feel like it's almost embarrassing to mention this, because it's so small compared to what workers go through," she said. "But I've had instances where I've ordered something online or bought something in the store, and I take it home, and I get a rash from it. And I take it back. As a consumer, you have the right to return something. But you know, as a worker I'm required to wear a uniform if I want to keep my job. If it's an irritant, or allergic response, it's much easier to associate that reaction to a garment. But if it's messing with your hormones, you probably wouldn't know," Anderson continued. "Why do I feel so tired? Why are my periods irregular? Why can't I get pregnant? Why is my hair so thin? You wouldn't think to tie that to a piece of clothing. It would be very difficult to prove."

There are compelling clues, however, that you and I are also victims of poisonous fashion. All we have to do is listen closely to our bodies and believe what they're trying to tell us.

CHAPTER 2

KILLER FASHION

How Scientists (Rarely) Measure
Chemicals in Our Clothes

Jaclyn gazed up at the doctor from her hospital bed. He was telling her she needed to sign a piece of paper authorizing the hospital to remove her colon. Her vitals were bottoming out; her organs were shutting down. He presented her with two choices: sign or die.

It was the second time in just a few years that she was at death's door. She closed her eyes and tried to tune in to what her body was telling her, using her Buddhist training. Perhaps she should simply surrender to what the doctor was saying. Perhaps she should accept what was happening instead of fighting the pain, the sharp knives shredding her intestines. Perhaps she should sign the paper.

How did she get here, to this bed, to this moment when her body, after years of crying out for her attention, had started shutting down?

In fact, it had been a slow process of tiny day-by-day exposures to fashion's toxic chemistry, as well as its toxic culture. The story starts decades before, when she was a girl in New Jersey.

The Steep Price of Cheap Clothes

I met Jaclyn through a bit of serendipity.

As I was looking into the question of what, really, is in the clothing we wear each day, I wanted to talk with people beyond those in the airline industry. If these unregulated chemicals are ubiquitous, they should be affecting other people, too, right? I had heard rumors about women in the fashion capital of New York having to quit their jobs after being exposed to chemical fumes from freshly arrived shipments one too many times. But I was unsure of where to start my search.

In the fall of 2021, the designer Arielle Crawford* invited me to give a video lecture, on whatever I wanted, to her class on sustainable fashion manufacturing at the Fashion Institute of Technology. Clearly, my lecture would be on toxic chemicals.

As I explained to the grid of faces on my screen my suspicions that fashion's chemicals are connected to chronic skin conditions and autoimmune disease, one face with the name Jaclyn volunteered the fact that she had worked in fashion and suffered from health issues. She didn't give many details. But after class, I asked Arielle for Jaclyn's email. Jaclyn agreed to meet up with me in her Brooklyn neighborhood. I thought she would just tell me about some nasty rashes. Boy, was I wrong. Rashes were just the start.

I spent more time and energy than usual fussing over my outfit that morning, mindful that I was about to have lunch with someone who, until recently, had worked for decades in fashion. When Jaclyn walked up to me outside the healthy café she had suggested, I noticed she was, indeed, way more stylish than me. Her fingers and wrists were crowded with vintage silver and turquoise rings and bracelets. A chunky Fair Isle cardigan framed a

---

*She's since retreated to the Texas countryside to be a self-sufficient and sustainable cowgirl.

cotton tee with faded lettering, and her jeans were artfully distressed. With shiny brown hair that waved gently to her shoulders, she had the kind of smooth, blemish-free skin—save a smattering of freckles—that makes you wonder what skincare products she uses. She looked younger than her forty-one years, impossibly cool.

But as we settled inside at a table to talk, I noticed that she held herself delicately, shoulders ever so slightly hunched forward, as if protecting herself from some unseen menace. As I was to find out, her overlapping illnesses and symptoms are invisible to strangers like me. I could only listen to this woman's story and, unlike so many doctors and even herself, believe what her body is trying to tell us.

Jaclyn grew up in the fashion industry—but not the glamorous side. Her father was a garmento, a clothing wholesaler, and she would go with him as a kid to visit the warehouses and thirteen ready-to-wear stores in New York and New Jersey that he owned. In high school (in the 1990s, around the time fashion production was furiously being outsourced to Asia), she learned to sew, making her own clothes. She didn't want to follow in her father's footsteps, however. She pursued a degree in fine arts at the University of Colorado Boulder, incorporating sewing into her art projects. When she graduated in 2003, she headed to New York, hoping to get a job in an art gallery. She papered the Chelsea arts district with her résumé, but she was only offered unpaid internships, which she couldn't afford to take. So she started applying to fashion jobs, figuring she knew the business well. It was supposed to be temporary.

That was how Jaclyn ended up in a dusty office in Midtown as an assistant to a small designer whose floral skirts and acrylic sweaters were sold in mass-market department stores. The office was dim, the little sunlight filtering through a few windows with metal blinds gone gray with dust. It was so crowded that Jaclyn had to ask her colleagues, all women at least twenty years her senior, to push in their seats so she could get to the bathroom. Fabric swatches covered her desk. At 5:00 p.m., after a day of opening boxes of samples straight from factories in India, she would run over to the Mercury Lounge or Bowery Ballroom to work the coat check and bar and hang out with indie bands. She didn't sleep much, but she needed both jobs to survive in one of the most expensive cities on earth.

After two years, she graduated to a high-end brand, designing coats. When she interviewed at an outdoorsy mass-market brand after that, the hiring manager asked her if she had ever considered overseeing production. "Your designs are so detailed," the manager said, and production does require a fastidious eye. It also pays better. Jaclyn took the job. Her dreams of working in the art world faded away.

With higher pay came higher stress. Every morning at that and the several jobs that came after, she arrived at the office to find up to 250 emails waiting for her from the other side of the world, alerting her to the status of hundreds of different garment orders in production. She became skilled at negotiating prices down while putting out metaphorical fires. One time, she got an email that a truck carrying fabric from a mill for an order (that was already on a tight deadline) had gotten in an accident, and now the entire shipment was at the bottom of a lake in China. All in a day's work.

As Jaclyn opened boxes of samples fresh from the factories, running her fingers over the fabrics and peering closely at the seams, threads, and trims to check for errors, the potent smell of chemicals assaulted her senses. The smell emanating from boxes from India and the boxes from China each had their own alarming odor. "I still have dresses from some companies that I have in ziplock bags because the smell is so bad," she said.

She received emails from third-party testing companies containing PDFs of up to twenty-four pages that assured her that the fabric samples were colorfast, didn't stretch out too easily, and didn't have certain azo dyes or other restricted chemicals. She didn't think much about it; it was just her job to check the tests before she could authorize shipment of the clothing. Not every brand she worked for bothered with these controls, however.

She also did factory visits. "I've had lots of weird factory experiences," she said. "I could show you pictures of the dye process, and these men, they're not wearing masks or anything." Especially in China, the fact that workers lived on-site, spending all their days and nights in the factory complex, disturbed her. One time she was doing a tour, heard a scream, and the electricity went out. Someone had been electrocuted. The tour continued, even as she pleaded to go check on the mystery employee. Worker injuries, she saw, were also all part of a day's work.

Life went on this way for six years, the same story at the next two brands, until 2012, when she started getting rashes on her arms and back. "I've always had weird skin issues, but it spiraled," she told me.

She went to get a patch test, wearing the square stickers of potential allergens on her back for a week—without showering, in the summer heat—with a visit to the doctor every twenty-four hours to check for reactions. When she got the results, she was dismayed.

At the café, she handed me a photocopy. There were plus signs filled for an azo dye ingredient, 4-Phenylenediamine, or PPD; ethyl acrylate, used to manufacture plastics and paints for textile coatings; and Azo Disperse Blue 106/124. Disperse dyes are used on synthetic fabrics like polyester. Each of these chemicals is common in the fashion industry (although the patch test didn't include all the thousands of chemicals that are used in clothing and textiles, only the fifty or so most well studied allergens that could fit on her back). And out of those fifty common chemicals, she was allergic to seven of them.

Jaclyn realized there could be hundreds or even thousands more triggers out there that she didn't know about. And unlike food, beauty products, or cleaning products, clothing doesn't come with an ingredient list. Even with her insider's knowledge of the industry and how clothes are made, Jaclyn felt as if there was nothing she could do to avoid those chemicals. Even if she quit her job, she had to wear clothing to live.

Not that she considered quitting. "I mean, I grew up in the industry," she said when I asked her why she didn't press the eject button then. "It's the only thing I knew or had done in my working career."

She felt helpless. So she ignored the results and kept going to work. "I mean, it was just a skin thing," she said. "This was like nothing compared to the health issues that came after that."

At the end of 2015, when she was about to go upstate for the Buddhist New Year's retreat she volunteered at every year, a sharp pain started in her gut. At first, it felt just like bad gas or constipation. But then it got worse, to the point where she could barely walk. Jaclyn had grown comfortable with ignoring her body, pushing it through, compartmentalizing her emotions and pain in order to show up for her obligations. She managed to get herself onto a bus and to the retreat.

As she sat in the kitchen on the first night, bawling, the chef put his foot down. "You have to go to the hospital," he said.

When she got there, they examined her and told her that her appendix had burst *four days* prior. When Jaclyn told me this part of the story, my jaw dropped. I remember the exact moment in 2017 when my appendix burst. I slid to the floor of the hospital waiting room, begging for help. I remember vomiting over the side of the cot and crying when they wouldn't give me morphine because I couldn't pee in a cup to prove I wasn't pregnant. Those seven hours before I was wheeled into the operating room were the most excruciating of my life. I couldn't believe she had gotten on a bus. I couldn't believe that she had *survived*.

She was transferred to a larger hospital in Albany, where they took the appendix out, but she refused to take oxycodone for the pain, fearing its addictive effects. She was back in the hospital a week later for an abscess.

After that, she went back to work.

The Dark Side of Bright Colors

About a year later, down in North Carolina, Professor Heather Stapleton bought a new polyester athletic shirt from a popular sports brand and took it home to her seven-year-old son. Her son has asthma, and as an environmental chemist and exposure scientist at Duke University's environmental policy division of the Nicholas School of the Environment, Stapleton was hyperaware of how easy it is to track allergens and chemical contaminants into the home. She usually washed all new clothing before letting her kids wear it, but on this day her son was in a hurry to put on his new shirt. So she relented, this one time.

Later that afternoon, he started complaining that he was itchy. When she pulled up his shirt, she saw that he had broken out on his back in the exact pattern of the black areas of the shirt. "That set my alarm bells off," she told me in early 2022. It reminded her of an article she had read about flight attendants getting sick, which had made her wonder whether the dyes in uniforms might be the issue. She then read a paper from a group of researchers at the University of Saskatchewan who had analyzed house dust and found brominated compounds, which are often associated with health problems in humans—some of the more toxic kinds of flame retardants, for example, tend to be brominated. But these weren't flame retardants in the house dust. The researchers thought they were some sort of brominated azobenzene disperse dyes, or "azo disperse dyes" for short.

Azo dyes are commonly used on all types of fabrics. They've gone from a gee-whiz technology of the industrial age to a cheap and ubiquitous ingredient in most modern fashion, making up 70 percent of the 9.9 million tons of industrial dye colorants used globally each year. And there's a special type of azo dye used on synthetic clothing called azo *disperse* dyes—as in, they are *dispersed* in a water-based solution for dyeing the polyester.

Stapleton wondered whether the substances the researchers found in the house dust were the same type of dyes that were in her son's polyester shirt. Luckily, she had access to world-class mass spectrometry equipment at Duke, so she could do what is called "nontargeted analysis."

Up until around 2010, environmental chemists, like those who work at the Environmental Protection Agency or the Consumer Product Safety Commission, couldn't just analyze a water or clothing sample and declare, *Here are all the things that are in it!* They needed to know what they were looking for. They needed samples of a substance, needed to know the chemical structure, and needed a hint that it might be toxic to even go to the trouble of testing for it.

But chemical companies are allowed by the EPA to keep the substances they're producing and selling a secret. "In 1998, for example, 40 percent of the substantial risk notices filed by manufacturers asserted the *identity* of the chemical was confidential," wrote Nena Baker in her 2008 book *The Body Toxic*. The EPA receives between fifteen hundred and three thousand notices per year from companies that they intend to begin manufacturing or importing a new chemical, and these notices are not required to contain any toxicity or exposure information. In 1998, the EPA found that only 7 percent of chemicals produced at high volumes came with all the data needed to assess their toxicity. Twenty-one years later, the EPA almost completely stopped posting substantial risk notices to the public at all, saying it didn't have the budget to replace the person who retired from staffing the website, and anyway, it wasn't legally obligated to do so. (They restarted the posts in early 2022 after an outcry.)

That leaves tens of thousands of chemical substances completely hidden from view. Your water (or clothing) could be swimming with toxic chemicals, but if scientists don't know they exist, they could never tell you that they're in there. They would just say there's no evidence that you're sick because of your water or clothing, even if you know in your bones (or your gut, or your skin, or your tight throat and watering eyes) that something is wrong.

But with high-resolution mass spectrometry, you don't have to wait for chemical companies to slip up and reveal what they're making. Nontargeted analysis allows scientists and researchers to play detective with a sample and see which chemicals are located inside. Which is what Stapleton did.

She brought the offending T-shirt to the lab, cut it up, and gave it to her colleague Dr. Lee Ferguson to analyze. Inspired by the Saskatchewan paper that pinpointed the presence of azo dyes in household dust, he had recently started looking more closely at these same azo dyes in other contexts.

"And sure enough, these halogenated disperse dyes were in that shirt," Stapleton said.

This was concerning. Some azo dyes are known skin sensitizers (which is the toxicologist's way of saying they can cause skin problems), but it's not the dyes themselves that cause the most serious harm. Many dyes release a basic chemical building block called *amines* when they come in contact with our skin bacteria. (We'll get more acquainted with the colorful history of these amines later.) And many amines are suspected to be carcinogenic, mutagenic, and genotoxic, meaning they could cause genetic changes in human cells, along with cancer.

Maybe azo disperse dyes shouldn't be on children's clothing.

As alarming as these results sound, the fashion and chemical industries have taken a more nuanced position on these dyes. First of all, some companies argue, it's only about 5 percent of all azo dyes that release these toxic amines. Second, the industry has (mostly) phased out these toxic types of azo dyes—though the European Union allows up to 30 ppm of restricted azo dye in any piece of clothing. Third, the industry maintains, too little of these amines would get into our bodies from fabric to cause us any harm. *It's not like you're eating your clothing*, an industry expert told me.

But if these azo disperse dyes are present in house dust—as these latest tests were showing—we *are* eating our clothing. This toxic azo dust isn't staying put on our garments. Rather, we're ingesting and breathing it on a daily basis, by virtue of the very fact that it's in our homes at all.

Stapleton and Ferguson wanted to confirm what they suspected: that the dyes in the house dust were from clothing, and that they could cause allergic reactions. And there happened to be an environmental analytical chemistry student who had a personal interest in how chemicals can contribute to allergic reactions looking for a PhD project.

Testing in Plain Sight

Kirsten Overdahl grew up in a medical family—her father is a physician. At eighteen months old, she was diagnosed with juvenile rheumatoid arthritis, an autoimmune disorder. She has also suffered from migraines and Raynaud's, the same condition my mom has, which involves loss of blood flow to the fingers and other extremities.

"I've always had an understanding of how much holistic health matters—not only what medicine can do, but the world that we're surrounded by, what's going into our bodies," she told me over video chat in March 2022, five months after successfully defending her thesis. Her understanding would only grow over time.

She had been reading about environmental justice and how people who live in poverty—and especially people of color in the United States—are more likely to live near toxic waste dumps and contaminated sites, to drink contaminated water, or to be poisoned by lead dust in their homes. As Harriet A. Washington writes in *A Terrible Thing to Waste*, environmental toxins have artificially depressed the intellectual capacity of marginalized communities in the United States. Black Americans and other people of color are more likely to live in "sacrifice zones," where their communities are drenched in hazardous chemicals.

Someone told Overdahl about the field of environmental toxicology, which looks at how everything we're exposed to can potentially affect our health. "It is easier to synthesize a new chemical than to regulate it," Overdahl said. It's estimated that there are between forty and sixty thousand industrial chemicals used in the United States that are untested for their effects on human health. "So it means that there's a lot of chemicals in commerce for which we just don't have information." She realized that she could use mass spectrometry to answer the questions that swirled in her mind and, more importantly, to make a positive impact on the world.

There was one big limiting factor to Overdahl's project: nobody had ever tested more than a handful of azo disperse dyes before. When the research team looked through the publicly available literature, they identified nearly five thousand chemicals with a chemical structure similar to azo disperse dyes being sold on the market. But very few were labeled as azo disperse dyes, or labeled at all. They were just chemical structures sitting in PubChem, the open-source database of chemicals and toxicity data that is managed by the National Institutes of Health, like, *Nothing to see here.* This black box made the chemical industry's claim that very few azo dyes are toxic seem ludicrous. More like: very few azo dyes have been tested and proven to be toxic. The rest? We, the consumers, have been led to believe that they are safe, despite having zero evidence to support the claim.

What's more, researchers had not even laid eyes on the vast majority of these commercial chemical products, much less checked to see whether they were safe to have against our skin. There were only eight lab-quality samples of azo disperse dyes, what are called analytical standards, commercially available for purchase in the entire world. Ferguson had already ordered some of them from a researcher in Brazil and an American chemical company to do his own analysis. Overdahl needed more.

"It was eye-opening. If I was a concerned citizen, and I thought I needed to be worried about azobenzene disperse dyes, there's no easy way to look that up," Overdahl said.

She would have to isolate, purify, and categorize the chemicals herself.

Another bit of serendipity aided the chemical detectives. It turned out that Ferguson's brother-in-law lives in High Point, North Carolina, next to the owner of one of the largest dye distributors in the United States. His brother-in-law put them in touch, and two weeks later, a box with little cans of dye showed up at the lab. Overdahl set to work hand-purifying the dyes down to their components—shades of red, blue, yellow, violet—to create lab-ready samples. That took her more than six months, and then another year to analyze them using high-resolution mass spectrometry to determine their structure. She was able to catalog twelve of them. Finally, after almost *two years* of painstaking work, she was ready to do some experiments.

Led by Overdahl, the research team bought thirteen pieces of polyester children's clothing from a local store and tested them. They found many of the same dye chemicals that were in the azo dye dust—the most commonly found one was Disperse Red 354— in both the name brands *and* the brandless items. One kid's shirt had more than 11,000 ppm, or 1.1 percent of the total weight of the shirt. That's three hundred times higher than the EU's limit for other azo dyes. When the team analyzed dust from 124 households with young children, they found azo disperse dyes in every single one. (This research should be published sometime in 2023.)

"Young children crawl around on the floor a lot, they put their hands in their mouths, and they ingest dust at up to twenty times the amount that an adult would ingest. Children still have developing organs and developing immune systems," Overdahl told me.

Stapleton was infuriated by the results. "We found these in baby pajamas. There could be a good proportion of kids that do react to them. And what does that mean for the lifetime risk factors for that child as they grow and develop? Can that lead to other diseases that are more severe, or more vulnerabilities to viruses and asthma and other skin conditions?" she asked.

That question wasn't just theoretical. It was very real to at least one mother several states away.

Keeping Our Kids Safe

In late 2021, I put a call out in my newsletter, looking for people who had experienced reactions to clothing, or whose children had experienced reactions. The responses flowed in, each pattern of overlapping health issues a unique fingerprint to that person and family.

I spoke to a mother in upstate New York whose toddler's reaction to clothing led her to realize the whole family had lead poisoning from their old farmhouse. I spoke to a woman who, after getting the Epstein-Barr virus, had developed fibromyalgia and become allergic to synthetic clothing. I spoke to an elderly Romanian immigrant to Alaska who suspects she had been poisoned by her workplace's carpet's fumes and now couldn't wear blue clothing without getting seriously ill. I spoke to a California marketing executive who was so allergic to disperse blue and black dyes that—before she realized and overhauled her closet—she would wake up bleeding, having scratched herself raw in the night. She still shops only at clothing stores with good return policies, in case a reaction shows up a couple of days after trying on a new piece of natural clothing.

I wasn't surprised by how easily I could find stories of allergic reactions to the clothes we buy in good faith and wear every day. According to the *Journal of the American Medical Association*, up to one in five people have experienced contact dermatitis, with itchy, flaky skin that can develop oozing or blisters. (We'll see that one-in-five number again.) The cause can be maddingly hard to pin down, since contact with a product as little as once a week can cause a constant rash, and sensitizing chemicals are so ubiquitous that you could encounter the offending substances in several different ways on any given day.

The issue is particularly acute for many people of color in the United States, and those who are economically disadvantaged. These individuals often live in frontline communities near toxic waste sites and manufacturing plants, where these chemicals are found not just in the clothes they wear but also in the very air they breathe and the water they drink. They often don't have the privilege of getting proper medical care that can help them pinpoint something they can then remove from their home. This systematic environmental racism is shameful. It also complicates research and reporting on the issue of chemical sensitivities to clothing—after all, how can you pinpoint the effects of one fashion-related chemical on someone when they are breathing in particulates and fumes from a highway cutting through their neighborhood?

To make a strong link between fashion and health for the purposes of researching this project, I realized I needed to find someone who otherwise had decent control over their environment, who had access to the medical system to aid in their sleuthing, and who—having tried everything else—finally realized it was the clothing that was the problem.

I found that person in Karly Hiser, a pediatric nurse practitioner in Grand Rapids, Michigan. When I got on a video call with her, she reminded me of the grown-up version of the type of athletic girl who played soccer at my high school, with long, dirty-blond hair pulled half back, no makeup, and a gray sweatshirt. Behind her, a pinboard was filled with Christmas cards featuring smiling families. She seemed a little bit nervous, her smile quickly fading into a frown as she told her story.

Her oldest son was two or three years old when his eczema got really bad. "Since I do work in the health-care field, I started doing research in my free time. And I noticed that eczema is increasing.

It led me down this path to think about what else is increasing in our modern-day world." Her conclusion? Chemicals.

She switched her family to fragrance-free soaps and nontoxic cleaning products like baking soda and vinegar, and cut dairy out of their diet, concerned about what cows are being fed. After baths, they would do something called "soak and smear," where they would cover their son head to toe in creams and Vaseline. "Everything we tried did not help," she said. The steroid cream he was prescribed irritated his skin more. Open wounds developed on his hands and behind his knees, and they got infected. "It was so hard to look at as a parent," she said.

Then, she started thinking about his clothing. "He's a really sweet, nice, low-key kid. And every morning getting dressed was a nightmare, just screaming tantrums." Like any parent on a budget, Karly had been buying cheap clothing from mass-market brands, including polyester athletic clothes. "I'm going to sound like a bad parent. But just anything I could find that was gonna be wallet friendly," she told me.

As her son got older, he finally had the words to describe what was bothering him. First it was the tags, and the seams.

Then, she finally realized, it was the clothing. All of it.

Desperate Measures

Fashion production manager Jaclyn's health spiraled downward. There was blood in the toilet every time she went. The gut pain started, and then became constant. She tried natural remedies and cut foods out of her diet. Neither helped. She went to one gastroenterologist who told her nothing was wrong, then another who was shocked. He said he had never seen someone so young with such bad Crohn's disease. She was thirty-five.

A few weeks after I met with Jaclyn, I saw an article by a Crohn's sufferer in the *New York Times* that I eagerly read and forwarded to Jaclyn. As the author said, doctors used to think that Crohn's, a type of inflammatory bowel disease, was caused by stress and diet. But according to the Mayo Clinic, many physicians now think these factors just inflame the symptoms, while the root cause lies in a combination of genetics and a malfunctioning immune system. In other words, it's another mysterious disease where the immune system, for some reason, has been prompted into overreacting and attacking its own body. A new theory posits that an intestinal infection—such as appendicitis—can allow allergens into the lining of the bowel, making the gut intolerant to whatever those substances are, usually foods.

If the lining of the gut is permeable to food allergens, I wondered when I read that, could it be possible that other substances could get in and cause mayhem, like fashion chemicals?

Jaclyn was always running to the bathroom at work. Once, she had an accident while on the subway train. Her doctor wanted to put her on Remicade, but her insurance wouldn't cover it. When she was at home, she was so weak that she would hold on to the furniture to get herself to the bathroom. "And, you know, I was still trying to go to work," she said. "I was trying to function normally, even though my body was shutting down."

She went to the doctor, and he told her she had to get to the hospital immediately. That is how she ended up weakly looking at a form that would have allowed doctors to take out her colon. Luckily, her father the garmento, who also has had serious digestive issues to the point of getting colitis (shared genetics or shared careers?), got on the phone with the doctors and told them to try the Remicade. Within twenty-four hours, her vitals had drastically improved, and she was out of the hospital ten days later.

The medicine allowed her to live her life, for a while. But she was still sick, and the nauseating ethics of her job were making her worse. Brands, as a matter of course, would just not pay the factories for orders, or they would stretch out payment for up to ninety days. "I was trying to protect the factories because I cared about them. I was flying overseas, and I'm sitting across from factory managers, it's Chinese New Year, and these women are crying that if I don't pay them, that factories are gonna shut down . . . The moral compromise of it was what was making me physically sick. It was traumatic. I'm working for a company that's causing them this harm."

I asked her which company. "It was various companies; there's lots of companies that weren't paying on time," she said. "I don't want to call out anyone in particular—it's a normal thing."

She was sick every time she came home from a factory, but she thought it was just the stress. One company she worked for changed ownership three times in the six months she was there, and the insurance changed with it. Every time that happened, she struggled to get her medication and treatment. But she couldn't quit because she needed the money. "It was a nightmare. I got to a point at one company where I was working to, like, four or five in the morning, getting home as the sun is rising, and sleeping for an hour." *What is the point of my life? I'm just working*, she wondered.

She developed itchy, painful psoriasis on her scalp. "It's something that people don't see, which is also like colitis or Crohn's disease. You're dealing with these, internal health issues, and you don't want to complain, but you're struggling." Then, her hair started falling out.

It's here in the story that she pulled a plastic bag out of her purse. Inside were dozens of individually bagged chunks of hair. "I know, that's so gross that I even have that," she said. "But it was just for my own sanity that I knew that this was actually happening." Someone in her Crohn's support group told her that her body was reacting to the Remicade, which at high doses is a chemotherapy drug. She didn't know what to do. "It's like, what's better—being bald or shitting my pants?" she said. She was switched to another medication, Stelara. Her hair started growing back, and the psoriasis mostly cleared up.

Meanwhile, at Duke, Overdahl was ready to take on the second half of her PhD project: figuring out whether all these azo disperse dyes could have the potential to be skin sensitizers.

Rather than force people to wear synthetic clothing, Overdahl did some test-tube work to show that the twelve azobenzene disperse dyes she had isolated bind to nucleophilic proteins, which is the first step in initiating a skin allergy. In short, yes, azo disperse dyes, and not just the ones commonly used in skin patch tests or the ones that have been phased out (supposedly) by the fashion industry, have that potential. And her experiments showed that the more dye there was in a piece of fabric, the more reactive it could be.

All the evidence pointed to an alarming situation: synthetic clothing is loaded up with azo disperse dyes that clearly have toxic potential—but we've barely scratched the surface about what they could do to various body systems. And children and adults are breathing them in and ingesting them daily.

Karly in Grand Rapids didn't know about this research—it would come out long after her son's skin crisis. At five years old, he was supposed to go off to kindergarten soon, but he refused to get dressed. "It was a little bit frightening to be like, *My kindergartener is gonna go to school naked!*" she told me. His aversion to clothes—the cheaper stuff from big-box stores that was laden with dyes and chemicals—was growing.

So she dragged out her grandmother's sewing machine from the 1950s, bought some supersoft, Oeko-Tex-certified, Tencel-cotton blend fabric from an eco-friendly online store, and made him some special underwear out of it.

It looked like, well, home-sewn underwear. But miraculously, it worked.

"I was shocked," she said. "He was like, 'Just clothe me head to toe in nice stuff.' So, now I make sweatpants, sweatshirts, and T-shirts. And he's a happy kid." Karly started making all her son's clothes from scratch, using this same fabric. In 2021, she found a manufacturer and launched a brand of nontoxic clothing for children called Crann Organic. It's been fun for her to include her son in running the business. She feels like they both have taken control of their health. His eczema, while it will probably never be completely cured, became manageable.

To be fair, Karly admits, her son's allergies extend to all sorts of things: mold, pollen, cats, dogs, and various foods, and he has asthma. "My suspicion is that he's probably a kid that was more likely to develop allergies . . . [and] that because of what he's exposed to in the environment, it's probably a bit worse," Karly said. He wheezes when he visits friends' houses where they use synthetic air fresheners. Karly herself had never used air fresheners because they gave her a headache. "But I never thought about why," she laughs ruefully.

"The issue I worry about is inhalation of fibers that have these compounds on them," Ferguson told me just a couple of months later. "I mean, is that contributing to asthma? Because, you know, skin sensitization is kind of the same reaction that you get when you have asthma; it's just one's inside your lungs and one's out on your skin."

I thought of Jaclyn, opening boxes with freshly finished synthetic fashion from Asia, day in and day out, her intestines writhing as her immune system attacked her own body, driven to a frenzy by some unknown substance.

As you can imagine, you need a special kind of dye that can bind to what is essentially plastic: polyester. When I asked Ferguson what safer alternatives to azo disperse dyes exist, he shook his head. "There's two chemical classes of disperse dyes," he explained. "There's azobenzene dyes [azo dyes], and then there's anthraquinone dyes. Those can be kind of toxic as well. So I'm not aware of any dyes that can be used to color synthetic fabrics that aren't risky from an exposure standpoint."

"That's a big statement," I said. "You're basically saying there is no safe dye for synthetic fabrics."

"I am saying that."

I sat back to consider this. All along, flight attendants and mothers and women who suffer from chemical sensitivity had been telling me that wearing synthetic fabrics made them sick. But I couldn't find any evidence that polyester or nylon was toxic. What if they were right all along? What if it wasn't the polyester or nylon or even the polyurethane fabric itself that was causing their adverse reaction?

What if, instead, it was the dye that was *on* them?

"Parents Aren't Ready to Hear It"

Stapleton, Ferguson, and Overdahl's work has opened the door for other researchers to pile into this emerging field of azo disperse dyes. Twenty-two azo dyes are banned in the European Union, but a 2020 study found their amines in half of the 150 textile samples researchers tested, and other research showed that in a quarter of the samples tested, they are present at high enough concentrations to be concerning for our health.

The French Agency for Food, Environmental and Occupational Health & Safety (ANSES) ran a biomedical study in 2018 that connected skin reactions in fifty patients to specific chemicals found in their clothing. In 2022, based on these results, it called for disperse dyes to be banned.

And yet, only a handful of researchers in the United States have any idea that this is a problem. And there's not enough research yet for a doctor or dermatologist to confidently apply this in their office.

"I do think that public demand can drive where research goes, and we're not necessarily having some of those conversations," Overdahl said. "But I think now somebody has asked, now it's time to start answering."

Even when parents come to the medical practice where Karly

works, asking for help with their child's eczema (and that happens a lot), they just want a quick fix. She knows that making home-sewn underwear can sound pretty radical to many people. Or even just paying more for clothes their kids will stain and tear and grow out of in a few months.

"Parents are not really ready to hear it," she said. "Changing your lifestyle and the chemicals you use takes a lot more work than ordering a cream."

It's not just safe clothes that are pricey. Research is also expensive. It costs money to run labs, to use equipment, to buy lab-quality samples, to hire researchers to do the work. It took Overdahl five years to purify, analyze, and test for only twelve dyes. The high cost of proving a chemical guilty—or even proving that it exists, that it's in our clothing, and that we're exposed to it—benefits the chemical companies and brands, which profit from keeping all this a secret. And all the while, universities and the government spend hundreds of thousands chasing evidence, and people spend thousands treating illnesses that they suspect—but can't prove—are related to the products they buy and put on their bodies.

Here's a good example. In 2008, hundreds of parents reported that their babies had developed horrific rashes from the heat-transfer tags printed on the inside of Carter's baby clothing. Parents described months of anxiety, bringing their newborns to the doctor and even the emergency room looking for answers. The Carter's CEO told a review blog that the company had tested the products and found "nothing in that label . . . that could cause that kind of irritation." Despite more than three thousand reports coming in by 2010, he concluded that it was a "rare allergic reaction in some babies with highly sensitive skin." Yet again, the fault was pinned on some overly sensitive bodies, letting the clothing off the hook.

But a 2011 lawsuit alleged that when the tags had failed the limit for infant clothing for phthalates, the Carter's team declared it a "PASS," and then said that moving forward, they would only be testing parts of the garment that a baby could put in its mouth. The lawsuit also alleged that the tags exceeded Carter's internal limit for formaldehyde. Carter's was likely doing only the legally required tests for the few substances that are regulated in children's clothing. There could be more lurking in the PVC tag paint.

The only gesture from Carter's toward taking responsibility was to offer refunds to parents who requested them. The Consumer Product Safety Commission didn't require a product recall.

In 2019, the advocacy organization Green America launched a campaign to get Carter's to institute a restricted substance list for its manufacturers, pointing out that in recent years, Carter's had reported to the Interstate Chemicals Clearinghouse's High Priority Chemicals Data System that it had used formaldehyde, arsenic, and cadmium in its products. Carter's finally published an RSL in 2020.

In 2008, hundreds of women joined a class action suit against Victoria's Secret, alleging that the bras gave them rashes so bad that, in some cases, they had permanent scarring. Tests of the bras found the presence of formaldehyde in some of them. Victoria's Secret's rejoinder was that it had its bras tested and they were either formaldehyde-free or had too little to cause health problems.

"It would be awesome if garment manufacturers labeled products containing trace amounts of chemicals (like formaldehyde) that are known allergens, just like they do with products containing nuts or eggs. But, until someone dies from a breast rash, it probably won't happen," a local newspaper columnist in California wrote in 2015 of her ordeal. A Victoria's Secret representative had contacted her to suggest she get a patch test and tell the representative what she was allergic to. Like Carter's before it, using this strategy of victim-body-blaming, Victoria's Secret emerged victorious—the suit was never even classified as a class action. (The brand might have heeded this warning and done some cleanup, though—it has since been named a leader in chemical management by the safe-chemistry industry group ZDHC.)

"I just find it frustrating that in my experience, we kind of stumble upon these potential problems by accident time and time again. We never know what these chemicals are," Stapleton told me. "When it comes to someone's health and particularly the health of a child or an infant, I think we need to be more transparent—in particular, chemicals used in products that come in direct contact with our skin and our bodies. If we don't, it's going to make it harder to understand what's contributing to cancer and asthma and all these other diseases that are out there."

Even Karly, a nurse practitioner, had to grope her way toward a solution. "You know, like the nutrition labeling for food, I would prefer if there was better labeling for clothing," she said. "It's hard to know what type of dye is used on something or if there's a chemical that was used in the finishing of it. Not all chemicals are bad or harmful, but I would like to at least be aware of what's in children's clothing."

Overdahl is similarly frustrated. "I see every day, just in our raw data that the instruments produce, that there are often thousands of chemicals in a sample that can't be matched to a known chemical. That's absolutely terrifying. This doesn't mean that every chemical is bad. Maybe it's harmless. But if we can't match a name to a chemical structure, it means that the data is not out there. So you can't say it's *not* safe, but you also can't say it *is* safe."

And, she adds, "Just because an individual level of a chemical is safe does not mean that all the chemicals in the aggregate will not have a certain consequence in the body. It is very, very difficult to study the effects of multiple chemicals at a time. As somebody who has navigated my own journey with immunocompromised conditions, it makes me realize that we can never just pin issues on one thing, right? We have to think in terms of systems."

I asked her if her work had changed the way she shops. "Honestly?" she said. "The biggest thing it's done is make me shop less."

When the pandemic hit in early 2020, Jaclyn was laid off. She had spent eighteen years in the fashion industry. She gave it everything: her mind, her body, her life. And it was over. Fashion had dumped her, just like it dumped factories that failed to meet the impossible deadlines, just like it dumped garment workers when they could no longer work the long hours in obedient silence.

Fashion did not care.

Outside the café, as we said our goodbyes, Jaclyn handed me a cotton net shopping bag she had tie-dyed herself. Then she asked me not to name any of the brands she had worked for. She wanted to keep the door open for applying to work in fashion again.

I felt like I was talking to a woman who had just described an abusive boyfriend, then told me she might move back in with him. I agreed to not name the brands, if only because it really didn't matter what the brands were. It is a systemic issue. It is normal. We are all swimming—and drowning—in fashion's toxic culture.

With all the complex chemical terms I've thrown at you, with the talk of faraway factories in countries with poor regulations, and synthetic clothing that's dyed with toxic colors, you might now be pining for a simpler time. Maybe a time before our fashion production was offshored, before synthetic dyes and synthetic fabrics made from fossil fuels were invented, before the Industrial Revolution even, when everything was natural and simpler.

But as I'm about to show you, fashion has *always* had a dark side. (Though it has admittedly gotten more complex, and more toxic.) I want to show you how we got here. So let's take a trip back in time.

PART II

A HISTORY OF CHEMICALS IN OUR CLOTHES

CHAPTER 3

TREACHEROUS TEXTILES

The Poisonous Price of High-Fashion Fabrics

We never do seem to learn.

Often, when I've told people that I'm writing a book about toxic fashion, they reach into the dusty cupboard of their mind, looking for something they can add, and they pull out the Mad Hatter. *Like how hats used to have a lot of mercury!* a typical conversation goes, the person shaking their head with a bemused smile at those crazy Victorians.

Well, the joke's on us. Because as those toxic trends have faded away, we've been busy coming up with new ways to poison ourselves with textiles and accessories. Almost always, it first becomes obvious that something is very wrong in the ateliers and factories where garment workers succumb to horrific illness. Whether something is done about it is a different matter.

Poisonous Rumors

Let's go back, about five hundred years, to the Renaissance and, more specifically, a June afternoon on which two notable women were out together shopping in the fashion capital of Paris, prepping for the August wedding of their son and daughter. It was a long time ago, so some accounts of this day differ, but according to Eleanor Herman's book *The Royal Art of Poison: Filthy Palaces, Fatal Cosmetics, Deadly Medicine, and Murder Most Foul*, the mother of the bride, who had lived in Paris since her own marriage, had been taking the mother of the groom, who was visiting from a kingdom south of France, to her favorite trendy boutiques to pick up clothing and jewelry for the big day. It was reported to be a tense shopping trip. As everyone knew, these two women had an intense dislike and distrust of each other. In fact, they were political and mortal enemies.

It was 1572, and the mother of the bride was Catherine de' Medici, the Florence-born Catholic queen mother of France. The mother of the groom was Jeanne d'Albret, ruler of Navarre, a tiny kingdom sandwiched in between France and Spain.

In another world, these women might have been friends and confidants, sympathizing with each other over cheating husbands, widowhood, and betrayals by power-hungry male rivals. But it was not to be. Jeanne was an enthusiastic convert to the protestant Calvinist religion—in direct opposition to Catherine's Catholic rule—and was a terrible scold when it came to fashionable luxuries. At age forty-three, she had the severe, straight-backed bearing that you would expect from a Puritan of her religious fervor, with little if any makeup to enliven her thin lips and sunken cheeks. She wore only a simple black mourning gown with white trim.

Catherine, on the other hand, was outgoing and artistic. She reveled in the pleasures of court life, including food and fashion. Paintings show her in dresses encrusted with rows of pearls and jewels. Her daughter, Princess Marguerite, was a beauty and a flirt who enjoyed a vast wardrobe of fancy clothes.

As the mother of the groom, Jeanne was expected to buy clothes for the bride. She also needed to buy some fresh items for her son, who was regarded as somewhat a country bumpkin by the Parisian sophisticates. Catherine hoped to smooth the way for a happy union between their two kingdoms—but Jeanne wasn't having any of it.

"Her face is spoiled by too much makeup, which displeases me," Jeanne wrote to her son, eighteen-year-old Henri, about his bride-to-be. Jeanne was in Paris preparing for the wedding, and her puritanical soul was offended by the Medici Catholic splendor on full display. "Although I knew it was bad, I find it even worse than I feared," she reported. "The men cover themselves with jewels. The king just spent 100,000 écus on gems and buys more every day."

The stress of the wedding negotiations was getting to Jeanne, and she was convinced that she was being spied on through a hole drilled in the wall of her apartment at the French court. "I feel that I may fall sick, for I do not feel at all well," she told Henri.

So here she was, spending a week being dragged from store to store in Paris by the domineering but fun-loving Catherine, or so the story goes. One store they dropped into was that of Catherine's loyal personal perfumer, Master René Bianco, a Florentine who had traveled with the teenage Catherine to France in 1533 for her marriage.

The Italians had a well-earned reputation as profligate poisoners. The Medicis themselves had set up factories to produce poisons, and the family's archives in Florence have letters with instructions on how to poison the wine and food of political rivals. The powerful Borgia family of fifteenth- and sixteenth-century Italy was rumored to have murdered rivals by placing poison not just in food and drink but in the pages of books, in flowers, and in gloves and clothing. All of them relied mainly on the heavy metals mercury, lead, antimony, and arsenic.

As the educated knew, the delicate art of mixing up a vial of perfume lent itself to the skill of making odorless but powerful venom. But Jeanne evidently did not believe in such frivolous rumors—at least, not at first. Inside the perfume shop in Paris, she must have perused the many scented objects, including gloves, holding them to her nose. Popularized by Catherine herself, perfumed gloves had become somewhat a necessary indulgence for those with means in this late Renaissance period. The gloves were dipped in boiled animal fat infused with jasmine, orange blossom, violets, musk, ambergris, and other herbs. The streets of Paris and even the inner courtyards of the palace were redolent with the smell of unwashed bodies and animal manure, and these gloves were a luxury to help protect the nobles' noses against the ever-present stench. (And mask the stench of the leather gloves themselves, as we'll see later.)

Jeanne eventually selected a pair for herself. By the time she arrived back at her royal apartments, she felt unwell and went to bed with a slight fever. Over the next few days, she developed an agonizing pain in her chest and had difficulty breathing. She died on June 9 in one final spasm of pain.

The word spread among European courtiers, according to Eleanor Herman's *The Royal Art of Poison*, that Catherine had deliberately poisoned Jeanne with the perfumed gloves. As a foreigner and merchant's daughter—albeit a fantastically wealthy one—Catherine had always been looked at with suspicion. Poisoned gloves, an exotic innovation infused with mortal sin, fit that narrative neatly.

Besides, everyone knew that when you were in a precarious position of power, you accepted gifts of fashion at your own peril. The myth of poisoned garments goes back almost as far as written history. In Greek mythology, Heracles is devoured by the flames of a poisoned robe. In seventeenth-century Indian mythology, the Mughal emperor Aurangzeb presented his rival's son with the gift of a *khilat*, an opulent honorary outfit, which dispatched him within the day.

But in the minds of the European royalty of the Middle Ages and Renaissance, poisoned clothing and accessories were not a myth but a very real danger.

Part of the predinner ritual for Louis XIV, which Herman

describes in *The Royal Art of Poison*, involved testers rubbing napkins, tablecloths, and dishes against their skin and kissing them to check for reactions. The servants who made King Henry VIII of England's bed every morning kissed every part of his bedding to prove they had not tainted them with poison. When garments arrived from the tailor for King Henry's son, Edward, they were washed and aired in front of the fireplace to remove any toxic substances and tested by a young servant to check for adverse reactions. The advent of germ theory being some way off, royalty would rather be handed used and soiled linens than take the risk of wearing a garment brushed with poison.

As for Elizabeth I, nobody but her most trusted retinue was allowed near her wardrobe. Her undergarments and "all manner of things that shall touch any part of her majesty's body bare" were guarded and closely examined before she put them on, according to a 1560 royal decree that Herman found, written by her loyal secretary of state, William Cecil. She was also not to accept any gifts of perfumed gloves or sleeves. It may have seemed like overkill, but twenty-seven years later, according to Herman, the French ambassador to England plotted to have one of Elizabeth's gowns poisoned, though the plot never seems to have been carried out except in Hollywood's imagination. (In the 1998 film *Elizabeth*, one of her ladies puts on a silk dress Elizabeth received from France and dies dramatically shortly after.)

Smearing heavy metal poisons of the day on cloth so they were absorbed cutaneously, or through the skin, would have been a decade-long murder plot, at least for an adult. But it turns out that the women of the European court *were* being poisoned—just by their own hand.

In the last years of her life, Elizabeth I deteriorated mentally and physically, becoming ever more paranoid that the Spanish Jesuits were plotting to assassinate her. She frequently threw temper tantrums, throwing her cosmetics and brushes at her ladies-in-waiting. Some experts believe her unstable last days were due to heavy metal poisoning from her lead-filled white makeup—a look often achieved through the use of mercury in the foundation, with a dusting of arsenic face powder on top. Queen Elizabeth died at the respectable age of sixty-nine, but she may have lived longer and with more equanimity were it not for the heavy metals piling up in her body.

As for Jeanne d'Albret, her autopsy revealed an abscessed lung, leading the surgeon to rightly conclude, "If her majesty had died, as it has been wrongly alleged, from having smelled some poisoned object, the marks would be perceptible on the coating of the brain, but on the contrary, the brain is as healthful and free from injury as possible." She likely died from a final bout of recurring tuberculosis, which could have been exacerbated by the stress of fighting with Catherine over the wedding.

There was no poison that, brushed on undergarments or gloves, could have dispatched its adult victim within days. Well, not yet. Such frightful substances would arrive centuries later, when fashion ushered in a new age of powerful fossil-fuel chemistry.

Until then, fashion did its murderous work slowly, through the casual and everyday use of heavy metals like mercury. Its most notorious victims weren't royalty but the underprivileged who labored in dusty and steam-filled workshops in service of the latest fashions.

Mercurial Hats

In 1857, a sixty-one-year-old hatter from Strasbourg, France, died by suicide by drinking a mercury-based hatting solution. For decades he had been breathing in mercury fumes and absorbing mercury through his cracked, bare hands as he created felted fur top hats for the men of the city to wear. Whether he made his decision after looking around at his colleagues and seeing his inevitable demise in their blackened teeth, swollen tongues, and trembling hands or because his severe depression and mood swings finally got the best of him, we don't know. Perhaps a bit of both.

His death came as no surprise to those familiar with the trade, writes Alison Matthews David in her deeply researched 2015 book *Fashion Victims: The Dangers of Dress Past and Present.* Europeans knew mercury was poisonous; government officials, doctors, and workshop owners had been wrangling over it for more than a century. Charles Dodgson, a.k.a. Lewis Carroll, published *Alice's Adventures in Wonderland,* with its trembling and illogical Mad Hatter, just a few years later.

But legislators were disincentivized to do anything about it. Hats were a core part of every man's wardrobe, and mercury was the fastest and most affordable way to create them. If a few working-class men had the shakes, well, life isn't fair, is it? Besides, how could you know those symptoms weren't actually because these men had poor lifestyle habits such as drinking? That was the argument from industrial hygienists of the day, anyway, eager to defend their friends the industrialists from any backlash or regulation.

For centuries, European men's hats—from the tricorn to the top hat and the tall-crowned capotain that we associate with the Puritans—were made of beaver fur. The fur was felted, or entangled, to form a thick, glossy, warm, and waterproof material. But the problem was that beavers were being hunted to extinction—first in Europe, and then in North America—and the supply chain was then disrupted by war. There was an alternative, cheaper pelt: the European rabbit. But there was a problem. Rabbit fur didn't naturally felt as well as beaver and needed to be broken down. Mercury made it possible, and it had the additional benefit of speeding up the process by four hours.

The hatters initially put up a good fight against the use of the heavy metal. The French hatters' guilds, a sort of protounion, outlawed mercury use in 1716, and mercury use in hat workshops was banned in Marseille, then Lyon and Paris. But by 1751, legislators had caved and legalized its use. Fast fashion was already forcing its way into Europe.

In 1757, as mercury-based hatting settled indelibly into Paris, a young French doctor named Jacques-René Tenon visited six hatting workshops in the city. Workers were "thin, feeble" and their hands trembled. They "sweat abundantly, coughed up viscous matter," and drank heavily to make it through the workday. One workshop that Tenon visited, Letellier's, had until recently used beaver fur boiled in untreated water, and still used a much more diluted mercury solution than other workshops. The workers in this workshop exhibited fewer symptoms, leading Tenon to recommend that hatters use less mercury or find a healthy substitute. Unfortunately, his writings went unpublished for almost fifty years.

But other doctors did start to take notice and published the things they saw. A five-month-old baby inhaled the vapor in a workshop and died. Hatters suffered convulsions and paralysis. In 1776, the *Gazette de santé* called mercury use "unnecessary, bizarre, and abusive."

This all raises the question of whether the men (and sometimes women) who wore these hats were also poisoned by mercury. There is no doubt the hats themselves were poisonous. When modern conservators at the Victoria and Albert Museum in London tested hats made between 1820 and 1930, one was 1 percent mercury by total weight of the fur felt. That's an astounding 10,000 ppm. (Modern brands try to keep mercury in fashion below .5 ppm, or twenty thousand times less.) Conservators are careful to wear gloves and masks when handling old hats today.

Matthews David points out that the furry exteriors of hats were often shellacked, and the interiors were lined with silk and trimmed with a leather hatband, likely protecting the wearer from direct, all-day exposure. But hats required frequent grooming and brushing to keep them glossy and neat, which likely sent mercury dust into the air. Women—wives and female servants—were the ones tasked to do it.

Would we know whether a nineteenth-century consumer was suffering from mild chronic mercury exposure? Its symptoms— fatigue, muscle weakness, rashes, gut pain, insomnia—can mimic other common conditions, such as autoimmune diseases, inflammatory bowel disease, depression, and other degenerative neurological conditions. To this day, there's no standard list of symptoms that can point definitively to mercury poisoning, and a victim of chronic mercury poisoning—with their mood swings, memory loss, mental illness, and suicidal ideation—can be written off as the town crank or drunk. A trembling, paranoid, grumpy woman was more likely to be called an old crone than be diagnosed with heavy metal poisoning.

There were a few labor organizing wins, although the use of mercury continued until astonishingly recently. In 1941, a year after *The American Public Health Report* discovered that 11 percent of hatters at five factories in Connecticut had chronic mercury poisoning, mercury use in hatting was finally banned in the state, and hatters switched to treating the fur with hydrogen peroxide.

But mercury in hatting was never officially banned in the UK. As late as 1966, there is a record of its use in British hat factories. The end of the Mad Hatter era came not with sweeping legislation but when men's hats, especially fusty felted fur ones, went out of style. The last hat factory in Danbury, Connecticut, closed in 1987, a victim of changing trends and globalization. Almost all fashion, not just hats, is now made abroad. But that wasn't always the case.

Playing in the Rainbows

Debbie sat in front of the laptop camera, using her long nails to carefully leaf through the death certificates on the desk in front of her.

"First walk me through your family's illnesses," I said. She exhaled. "If you need a moment or don't want to talk about something, that's okay," I quickly added.

"No, I'm an open book," she said. "Because people need to know." She began listing them out. Debbie's paternal grandfather, who worked in a tannery, had prostate cancer, and her father was diagnosed with the same two years earlier. Her other grandfather on her mother's side had colon cancer. Her paternal grandmother had chronic heart failure, and her great-aunt had heart disease. Her older cousin and cousin's daughter both passed away from breast cancer. Her younger brother had just suffered a health emergency at age forty-two that the doctors thought might be a heart attack. Her mom had early-stage colon cancer and had cysts in her breast removed.

She peered at the certificate for another great-aunt who had heart disease and diabetes. "It says cancer, I can't make out the rest," she said, sighing. She pulled another one out of the pile. "My aunt—my father's sister—is the only one whose death certificate says 'Cause of Death: Natural.' But she also had COPD." Chronic obstructive pulmonary disease. "We figured that was from smoking."

I first read about Debbie in the *Times Union*, a local upstate New York newspaper. (God bless local newspapers!) The author, Brianna Snyder, wrote the 2016 investigation into the many toxic waste sites in Gloversville, New York. I found her on Twitter and asked her if she could connect me to Debbie (a pseudonym; she's well known in the community and fears these news stories might impact her work in health care). Within a week, I was on a video call with this forthright woman.

Debbie was born and grew up in Gloversville, the erstwhile capital of leather accessories, about fifty miles northwest of the state capital in Albany. Leather making is in Debbie's blood: her grandfather, mother, and uncle all worked in the tanneries in town.

What also might be in her blood are, quite literally, the chemicals used to tan and dye leather. In Gloversville's glory days, in the late nineteenth and early twentieth centuries, two million gallons a day of tannery waste, including animal fat and flesh and tanning chemicals, poured directly into the Cayadutta Creek, which changed colors daily according to the dyes used. As it flowed through the backyards of Gloversville residents, ten-foot-high hummocks of noxious suds piled on the oily water.

"As kids, we played in the creek," Debbie said, shortening the *ee* in *creek* to "crick." "We thought it was cool because it was rainbows. When you look back now, it was all the toxic chemicals. And we're playing in the rainbows, catching crawdads and whatever else was in there."

Leather tanning has always been a foul and unhealthy process. For hundreds of years, tanneries reeked not only of rotten flesh but also excrement. Many tanneries in Europe used dog, chicken, or pigeon manure to preserve the hides and make them soft and pliable. Some traditional tanneries in Morocco still use excrement to this day. Tanners could also substitute high-tannin materials like bark or chestnuts for urine, but that yielded a thicker, less pliable leather, better for stiff dress shoes than supple accessories like gloves (and that vegetable-matter tanning process took more than a year).

The element chromium was discovered in 1797 by the French chemist Nicolas-Louis Vauquelin, and it almost immediately upended the centuries-old process of preparing leather for commercial use. By the mid-1800s, manufacturers had discovered that using chrome salts instead of traditional tannic substances sped up the tanning process to just a day, yielding a supersoft, thin, and comfortable leather that held on to bright colors—a real benefit since chromium turns leather blue until it is dyed. It also yielded products that didn't smell like a latrine.

Around that time, in 1853, a hamlet called Stump City in New York State, population 1,318, incorporated and changed its name to Gloversville. It had big plans to become a hub for high-quality leather gloves, and when the railroad came through in 1870, business boomed. About 90 percent of gloves sold in America between 1880 and 1950 were made in the so-called Glove Capital of the World. In the 1890s, stately Victorian mansions sprouted up in town, built by what people said was the highest per capita population of millionaires in America.

Outside of the ornate foyers of the wealthy, however, Gloversville was not the most pleasant place to live. The creek was devoid of life. There were reports of asthma and other respiratory problems, and residents said they could light their tap water on fire.

"They said our city smelled so bad because of all the chemicals, but nobody complained because everybody had money," Mayor Dayton King told the science publication *Undark* in 2017. Those chemicals included formaldehyde and chromium.

Debbie was born at the local hospital in 1967, and except for maybe three years in her early childhood, she's spent her whole life in Gloversville. The first sign that something was off was when one of her classmates died of leukemia in second grade, and then another in third or fourth grade, as Debbie remembers it. Then Debbie got her period on the early side, at age ten. "I noticed that happens a lot around here, where the girls tend to start their cycle early," she said. It presaged a lifetime of fertility and menstrual problems.

When Debbie was in middle school, cheaper foreign labor began to chip away at Gloversville's dominance, moving glove-making to places like Kolkata, India. Fake leathers like PVC started winning the hearts of fashion brands. Still, she and her friends wore a lot of leather: leather pants, leather jackets and coats, leather purses, and leather gloves. "I would take the pants off and the dye would be on my skin. I had to take a shower to get it off," she said.

By the 1980s, when Debbie was in high school, the Clean Water Act had forced tanneries to install wastewater treatment systems to mitigate the effects of the chromium-laced effluent. But many couldn't afford the million-dollar price tag, and they shut down, decimating the local economy. Only a few tanneries survive today, focused on luxury custom-leather products and military dress gloves.

But the contamination remains. Almost thirty EPA-designated sites around Gloversville are known or suspected to be toxic. The way locals tell it, a panoply of illnesses—neurological disease, cancer, and respiratory issues—seem to stalk the community.

Debbie has worked on and off as an administrator in several health centers that provide dentistry since her first job in the late 1980s. And from the beginning, she was alarmed by the number of rotting teeth she saw in local kids. "You can't tell me it's just from them not brushing their teeth," she said. Decades later, her own granddaughter would get surgery to remove six rotten teeth. Another job had her administering contracts for an insurance company. As she perused the addresses listed for young people with mental illness, she was alarmed by what seemed to her a cluster of diagnoses she saw in Gloversville and the nearby neighborhoods: depression, schizophrenia, bipolar disorder. She's not an epidemiologist, so she could very well be off in her assessment. But all these observations together were enough to stop her from drinking from the tap, and start buying bottled water.

That was twenty years ago. Even with her precautions, her own health troubles have mounted. She had multiple surgeries for endometriosis and four miscarriages—three before and one after having her only child, a son. By the time she was diagnosed with cervical cancer, she had given up on trying to have more kids and decided to get a full hysterectomy and one of her fallopian tubes removed. Her sister also has cervical cancer, which recently came back after remission. Debbie has had several cancerous moles removed, and she's chronically tired and in pain. Her doctor thinks it might be fibromyalgia. Her granddaughter's mother also has fibromyalgia.

Chronic chromium VI poisoning, according to the CDC's Agency for Toxic Substances and Disease Registry, presents itself most often as respiratory ailments: sinusitis, nasal septum perforation (holes in the cartilaginous wall between the nostrils), bronchitis, asthma, rhinitis, and lung cancer. When I told Debbie, her eyes got wide. Her grandfather had emphysema. Another aunt had "Respiratory Arrest" listed on her death certificate. Her mom has asthma, and Debbie has developed it, too.

"Perforated septum . . ." she mused. "Does a deviated septum count?" At one point her neighbors told her she snored so loudly they could hear her from across the yard when her windows were open. Her classmates have been posting on Facebook about getting sleep studies and whether they want to give in to getting a CPAP machine, which they call a Darth Vader mask, to aid in respiration at night. "I do Flonase at night, and I take another Zyrtec, and hopefully, you know, I wake up in the morning." She shrugged.

I asked Debbie if she ever has reactions to certain products. "Perfumes," she said without hesitation. "Sometimes candles. Painting a wall will definitely set me off. My asthma kicked up when I got this new furniture, and it's cloth. I went furniture shopping with my mother, and I immediately filled up"—what she calls getting congested—"when I walked in." She's broken out in hives due to certain makeup brands, body washes, dish detergents, and laundry detergents.

I asked her: "What about clothes?"

"Yes." She nodded. "People think I'm crazy. But I can take an item off of a hanger and I can smell the chemicals in the clothes. I can't buy it. I can't try it on. It repels me. I don't know if it's because I grew up around here. The smell of the tanneries is . . . indescribable. There's nothing that compares to it. I just got into a habit that every time I buy something new, I always wash it first before I wear it because I would put something on, and I would be itching all day. I'd itch myself raw."

A light bulb had gone off in her head about her intolerance to chemicals. "I just figured it was me," she said. "I didn't know it was, you know, a result of *this*." She waved her hand to indicate everything around her.

Unfortunately, even though it's obvious to Debbie, it can never be definitely proven what might have caused Gloversville residents' chronic and compounding illnesses because of the variety of chemicals poured into Gloversville's water and air from so many different businesses. But who would Debbie or anyone else sue, anyway? It's not like one large company came in and caused this. All the small tanneries are long gone, bankrupt, their owners themselves sick or long dead.

"I don't get mad," Debbie said. "You can't blame our parents. You don't know what you don't know. Back then, nobody even thought about what these chemicals could do. They were just trying to make a living. I think that's the mentality of a lot of the people around here."

But people know now. It's just that tanneries are located in countries where, like Gloversville sixty years ago, the smell of money is stronger than the smell of chromium. When I asked Debbie if she knows that Europe will recall, and in some cases destroy, gloves with too much hexavalent chromium on them, she was surprised. "Wow," she said.

I didn't have the heart to tell her that no one is doing the same in the US. While Europe puts a limit on the level of chromium that can be in consumer products, our federal government does no such thing. In fact, I would later see this for myself in a pair of gloves I purchased from a large mall brand, which were infused with incredibly high levels of chromium.

Before you swear off leather and switch to vegan fashion, however, I have bad news for you.

Space-Age Fabrics for Modern Life

As fashion-production techniques evolved, so, too, did the chemicals used. No longer content to merely wrest natural fibers into submission, chemists entering the twentieth century turned to making fabrics themselves out of fossil fuels—fabrics that would fit the needs and specifications of a modern (yet still brutal) world.

Polyurethane, also known as PU, which is often marketed as a vegan alternative to leather, was invented in Nazi Germany in 1937. One of its first uses was for mustard gas–resistant garments. DuPont started promoting its nylon for stockings in 1939 by saying it was made from "coal, air, and water." (At the 1940 New York World's Fair, Miss Chemistry emerged from a test tube wearing DuPont's synthetic fibers, like a plastic party surprise.) Polyester followed in 1941, acrylic to replace wool in 1950, and spandex in 1959.

But PVC came before all that. In 1926, Waldo Lonsbury Semon, an American researcher at the B. F. Goodrich Company, took a seemingly useless material called vinyl chloride and added a solvent, accidentally creating a flexible plastic called polyvinyl chloride. The polymer was used first to create golf balls and shoe heels but, with some tweaking of the recipe, would go on to be present in shower curtains, raincoats, and all sorts of pleather fashion.

By 1959, industry scientists were concerned about PVC's toxicity, especially when it came to the factory workers who made it. A study on rabbits repeatedly exposed to vinyl chloride showed worrying cell changes that indicated it was carcinogenic. "We feel quite confident . . . that 500 ppm is going to produce rather appreciable injury when inhaled 7 hours a day, five days a week, for an extended period," a Dow Chemical toxicologist wrote privately to his counterpart at B. F. Goodrich. "As you can appreciate, this opinion is not ready for dissemination yet and I would appreciate it if you would hold it in confidence but use it as you see fit in your own operations." B. F. Goodrich saw fit to ignore it.

British designer Mary Quant was the first designer to use PVC, in her 1963 Wet Collection. The mod designer said she was "bewitched" by "this super shiny man-made stuff and its shrieking colours." Her shiny raincoats and hats ended up on the cover of *Vogue* and on celebrities like Cynthia Lennon. Paco Rabanne, André Courrèges, and Pierre Cardin quickly followed with their own PVC creations: skirts, over-the-knee boots, gloves, and clear raincoats that evoked excitement around the space age and the wonders of chemistry.

Wonders of chemistry, indeed. By the mid-1970s, clusters of a rare liver cancer were showing up in PVC plant workers as well as in rodents exposed to vinyl chloride, but the PVC industry managed to delay the release of the data. When five PVC plant workers died in Louisville, Kentucky, the media pounced. The rat was out of the lab, so to speak, and the US Occupational Safety and Health Administration (OSHA) dropped the allowable exposure of vinyl chloride in PVC factories from 500 ppm to 1 ppm. Industry spokespeople warned that US plants would have to close, but within two years, they had all met the new standard, and PVC production continued to increase.

It's not just workers who are exposed to vinyl chloride, though. PVC plastic off-gasses—breathes out into the surrounding air—vinyl chloride over its entire lifetime. But the fumes are worse when it's new. In fact, part of that seductive "new car smell" is vinyl chloride fumes.

A 1979 scientific review by the International Agency for Research on Cancer (IARC) found that "there is no evidence that there is an exposure level below which no increased risk of cancer would occur in humans." In other words, there is no safe level of vinyl chloride.

The industry responded by secretly funding a competing scientific review, pressuring researchers to retract any study linking vinyl chloride to cancer, offering the EPA its own data to "help" with its risk assessment, and securing spots for industry members on the EPA's risk review panel. In 2001, after fifteen years of work, the EPA published its new assessment of the risk of cancer stemming from vinyl chloride exposure. It was ten times lower than the previous assessment. "As a result, allowable pollution levels may increase by 10-fold," wrote Jennifer Beth Sass, Barry Castleman, and David Wallinga in their 2005 scientific review, "Vinyl Chloride: A Case Study of Data Suppression and Misrepresentation."

The EPA also said that the only risk from vinyl chloride exposure was for liver cancer. All that other data connecting vinyl chloride to brain, lung, and even mammary cancer? Not relevant.

It should be noted, however, that the EPA does not govern what is used in or on consumer products. That falls to another underfunded federal agency, the Consumer Product Safety Commission, which we will talk about in another chapter.

In the 2010s, another issue hit the headlines. PVC is a hard plastic unless something is added to make it pliable. That something is most often phthalates, which are endocrine disruptors, and reproductively toxic. This tends to manifest in baby boys born with swollen scrotums and, in rare cases, undescended testes and abnormal urinary openings. Research has connected phthalates with reduced fertility in men, and studies have also linked these chemicals to asthma, cancer, and behavioral problems in children of all genders.

The "regrettable substitution" shuffle started. Producers of thousands of products replaced one phthalate, DEHP, with another, DINP, which scientists then discovered is correlated to male genital birth defects and damaged adult male fertility. In response to the fears of parents, the CPSC banned phthalates from use in some children's products in 2017, while still allowing PVC in children's products. But advocacy groups are still finding phthalates in children's bags and sandals today.

Thoroughly Modern Cotton

While some scientists were devoting themselves to creating entirely new, man-made fabrics, others were attempting—with the modern miracle of chemistry!—to improve the ones that already existed.

Ruth Benerito was born Ruth Rogan in 1916 to a progressive New Orleans family. Her mother was an artist and encouraged her children to follow their dreams, while her father emphasized the value of education. Ruth rose to the occasion, enrolling in Newcomb College, Tulane's women's college, at age fifteen.

"We didn't have the women's movement and any of those things going on at the time. My good friend and I were the only two [women] that were allowed to go to the Tulane campus to study physical chemistry," she said in a 2002 interview. When she graduated, she had a hard time finding work. The country was still in the throes of the Great Depression, and one of the only careers available to women was teaching. She found a job teaching science, math, and driving safety outside New Orleans. "I was the first driving safety teacher in the state of Louisiana, but I didn't know how to drive," she said. "One time I even went forward into the ditch."

Undeterred, she took night classes at Tulane to earn her master's degree, then received her PhD from the University of Chicago. In 1950, she married Frank Benerito and began working at the Southern Regional Research Center of the US Department of Agriculture (USDA), where she was tasked with saving the cotton industry.

In the 1960s, cotton still made up three-quarters of the textile market. It can be processed into a versatile natural fabric that is useful for everything from sheets to canvas shoes to sundresses, which is why it had been a staple textile for centuries. But raw cotton fibers are made of cellulose, a material with a weak, chain-like

structure very prone to wrinkles, so it had become increasingly un-
popular with the growing cohort of middle-class women who
made the purchasing decisions for their households. These
modern, postwar housewives couldn't afford full-time help, and
they didn't want to spend all their time ironing their family's
clothing. As options for fabric increased, more and more women
were choosing wrinkle-free clothing items made of the latest synthetics.

Wrinkle-resistant clothing wasn't brand-new for this generation. Before the 1960s, you could buy wrinkle-resistant cotton
clothing treated with chemicals like formaldehyde, which worked
by strengthening the bonds and setting them into a permanently
flat configuration. But the finish made the fabric incredibly brittle,
and consumers were noticing. "You could sit down, and your shirt
would rip across the back," Noelie Bertoniere, a former colleague
and friend of Benerito, told *Chemical & Engineering News* in 2013
of the early wrinkle-free fabrics. And when you tried bleaching the
formaldehyde-laden cotton with chlorine, and then ironed it, the
fabric would yellow. Not great for white button-downs.

Benerito's team was put on the task of finding a better wrinkle-
free fabric, and they eventually discovered the superior cross-linking
properties of dimethylol dihydroxyethylene urea (DMDHEU).
(According to her colleagues, Benerito was always careful to give
credit for the scientific advance to her team instead of hogging it
for herself.) DMDHEU made it possible to "permanent press" cotton without making it too stiff or brittle. And using her method,
the textile industry gleefully attached all sorts of performance
chemical products to cotton—flame retardants and stain repellents
being two popular ones, but also antimicrobials, anti-odor finishes,
and anti-shrinkage finishes.

Benerito's work is credited with saving the cotton industry from
complete ruin. The USDA turned the formula over to America's
cotton industry, and it spread quickly through the textile mills of
the South. Polyester ended up taking the lion's share of the market

anyway—it accounts for more than half of fashion textiles today. But without all these performance finishes, cotton might have ended up like linen, a formerly beloved fabric that now is associated almost exclusively with artfully wrinkled farmhouse bedding and makes up less than 6 percent of the global market.

The problem is, when DMDHEU breaks down, it releases one of its ingredients: formaldehyde. Although formaldehyde naturally occurs in small amounts in places as diverse as the human body and apples, as the dose grows, it quickly becomes dangerous. We can smell it at the level of 1 ppm, which is also where it starts causing eye, skin, and lung irritation. At higher doses, it is carcinogenic.

This is a theme with fashion chemistry. While the chemical used on a textile might not in itself be dangerous, over time it can break down into its toxic ingredients. So that ingredient—whether it's formaldehyde in no-iron trousers or an amine in a dyed shirt—might poison garment workers, then contaminate the local community, and then, after a brief sojourn as a harmless performance substance on your fashion, show up again to be breathed in or absorbed by your skin in small amounts, day after day.

They Don't Care

In 1981, Americans saw a minute-long TV commercial in which women held dripping ice cream cones and danced across the screen in soiled pastel blouses, joyfully singing "I don't caaaaaaaare!"

"Care-free Visa releases stains and dirt in the wash," a female voice narrated as the women cross-stepped behind a giant washing machine. "And Visa resists wrinkles!" In other words, Visa (not to be confused with the unrelated credit card company) was an "easy-care" fabric, bringing convenience to millions of women who hoped that—with the help of modern chemistry—they could finally step out of the laundry room and have it all.

In the early 2000s, there were at least nine textile companies with more than $1 billion each in revenue in the US. Today, only one remains: Milliken. It has survived by transforming from a textile company that also makes some chemicals into a chemical company that also happens to make some textiles. Milliken & Co. has never willingly shared any of its financials. But Visa fabric is still a core part of a business that, according to a Forbes estimate, made Roger Milliken, CEO and heir to the family business, one of America's richest men and a billionaire four times over by 1989.

Since its founding in 1865 in Maine as Deering Milliken & Company, purveyor of wool and dry goods, the company has managed to ride each wave of US textile manufacturing before it crested and broke. In 1884, long before the decline of New England's textile empire, the founder, Seth Milliken, jumped into the South's cheaper, less unionized labor pool by building his first southern plant in South Carolina. In 1957, Deering Milliken got in on synthetics with Agilon, a stretchy fabric for women's hosiery. That same year, Roger Milliken established Milliken Chemical as its own business unit.

In the 1960s, roughly 95 percent of America's fashion was still manufactured domestically. By the 1970s, that number was already starting to shrink. The Clean Water Act of 1972 gave American chemical manufacturers, dyehouses, and textile finishers further incentive to move offshore. When the North American Free Trade Agreement came into force in the early 1990s, there was no longer any reason or incentive to manufacture fabric in the United States. Fabric can be made and dyed cheaply in almost any developing country that has somewhat reliable electricity, an ocean port, and people desperate enough to work in harsh conditions for as little as fourteen dollars a month. Roger Milliken, a staunch Republican, came out against his conservative allies by funding a pugnacious campaign to protect American manufacturing. But he couldn't fight the tide. The textile and apparel sector lost 76.5 percent of its jobs between 1990 and 2012.

Textiles are cheap. But the chemistry that imbues fabric with performance qualities? That is something else. Chemistry can have name recognition—Milliken's Visa fabric and 3M's Scotchgard are two examples. Chemistry can be a trade secret, its true composition and potential health effects obscured from the government and consumers for decades. Plus, chemistry can be patented, and thus marked up in price.

Even though they are largely invisible to you and me, fabric finishes have become a core part of textiles. A 2012 report from the German Federal Institute for Risk Assessment estimated that "the residues of finishing agents in garment textiles may account for up to 8 percent of the textile product weight."

Researchers are even discovering that microfibers from natural textiles like cotton aren't breaking down as quickly as we thought when they hit waterways, potentially because they are so thoroughly coated in chemicals and polymers.

"Companies increasingly started prioritizing function in marketing," said Muhannad Malas, who was a campaigner against toxic chemicals in consumer products for six years in Canada before he joined the fashion team at the climate advocacy organization Stand.earth.* "A lot of companies have been developing products that provide a certain type of function and then use that function to promote their product. And that happened at the expense of public health and the environment, because often they were using chemicals that were not well studied, sometimes not even studied at all."

Fabrics coated with a secret recipe of chemicals and marketed with high-performance qualities are almost the only kind of fabric that can carry a price high enough to support American wages, workplace safety, and environmental controls. Of course, that

---

*He has since left Stand.earth and is now the law reform director for the Canadian charity Ecojustice.

doesn't guarantee performance finishes are safe, even when they are manufactured here, under the distracted eye of the EPA.

A study published in the 1980s of people who worked at three unnamed permanent-press garment factories in Georgia and Pennsylvania in the 1950s through the 1970s showed that they were at high risk of developing several different cancers. In 2004, a follow-up showed that at exposures as low as .15 ppm, workers were at a higher leukemia risk.

In 2010, when more research showed formaldehyde exposure could cause cell mutations and low red blood cell count similar to those caused by benzene, regulators started taking notice. "If somebody were to tell me they've got a new chemical, it's great for keeping your lawn green or whatever, and by the way, it seems to cause these low blood counts, I would say don't even go near it, don't manufacture that," Bernard Goldstein, a former dean of the University of Pittsburgh School of Public Health and assistant EPA administrator for research and development from 1983 to 1985, told PBS *NewsHour*.

The Government Accountability Office, the investigative arm of Congress, tested 180 items of clothing and bed linens and found that about 5 percent of the items tested, including a boy's baseball cap and crib sheets, had formaldehyde levels above 75 ppm. (The US doesn't have federal limits for formaldehyde on adult clothing, so they were tested against Japan's standard, which is the most stringent.)

This result—most stuff is okay, just try to avoid easy-care button-downs—seemed to placate the public, and the subject of toxic wrinkle-free cotton faded from headlines.

Meanwhile, Milliken & Co. had not only survived the Great Offshoring, it thrived, going into carpets and colorants, buying up bankrupt and struggling textile mills and chemical companies, and opening outposts in Asia and Europe. It amassed more than twenty-three hundred patents on compounds that give fire retardancy to fabrics, stain repellency to tablecloths, and chemical protection to lab coats. Though, ever on top of trends, it released a formaldehyde-free upholstery fabric called Breathe in 2017.

In 2018, tensions flared again when the EPA was rumored to be holding on to a report that said low levels of exposure to formaldehyde puts workers at risk for leukemia. The American Chemical Association funded competing research to muddy the waters, essentially showing that not *all* people who were exposed to formaldehyde had health effects, and then said the data the independent researchers was finding was "weak and inconsistent."

In April 2022, the EPA finally released a draft risk assessment of long-term formaldehyde exposure, saying that there were demonstrable links at low doses to nasopharyngeal cancer, myeloid leukemia, and sinonasal cancer, plus a reasonable certainty that it's also linked to allergies, asthma, and male and female reproductive toxicity. As of October 2022, it still hadn't finalized the draft after the comment period.

Anyway, the EPA has got even more pressing—and more high-profile—chemicals on its regulation docket. Like PFAS.

Forever Chemicals

In 2014, Milliken bought an old textile plant in Georgia called King America Finishing, owned by the Chicago-based Westex, which manufactured fire-retardant and water-repellent performance fabrics. The factory had a sordid past. In 2011, the worst fish kill in Georgia's history—thirty-eight thousand dead fish over a seven-mile stretch—started right below its wastewater pipe.

Even after Milliken revamped its wastewater treatment system, in the three years leading up to the fall of 2020, the plant in Georgia was noncompliant every single reporting quarter, paying the state $83,000 in fines for violating the federal Clean Water Act by dumping toxic effluent in the Ogeechee River. That's not much money for a company like Milliken, but on its glossy corporate sustainability website, it said one of its environmental goals is to have zero violations. One way to reduce your violations is to bring your pollution down below limits. Another way is to increase the pollution limits. A third way is to get rid of testing altogether, so nobody knows whether you're over the limit. So in September 2020, Milliken put in a request for a new permit that would increase the limits on pollutants it discharges into the river as well as reduce the frequency of water-quality tests. Plus, it wanted the testing for formaldehyde and THCP, an ingredient chemical for flame retardants, eliminated.

This astounded the Ogeechee community. "I was literally born and raised on the Ogeechee. My parents brought me home from the hospital on a boat," one woman said at an online public hearing, trying to keep her voice from cracking. "My children cannot enjoy the river in the way I did growing up, and that seriously breaks my heart. If this company cannot meet the minimum requirements of this stringent permit, why are we lowering the minimum to the detriment of the public and the people who want to enjoy the river?" She gathered herself. "If there's not a standard, create a standard."

Five local community members spoke out against the relaxed permit and against Milliken. Nobody from Milliken was there to defend the company or its application.

But there was a new chemical in the mix that the draft permit didn't mention: PFAS. "We know the facility is discharging significant amounts of it," said Damon Mullis, executive director for the nonprofit Ogeechee Riverkeeper, at the hearing. "We know at this point that fish in the river are contaminated. And we also know it has very serious health effects."

The American chemical company 3M invented the chemical compound perfluorooctanoic acid, or PFOA, in the late 1940s. 3M started selling PFOA to DuPont to use in Teflon nonstick pans and other products. (Until the late 1990s, its sister chemical, PFOS, was the main ingredient in 3M's Scotchgard, the popular spray that stainproofs textiles.) Unlike other exciting advancements in chemistry, 3M didn't publicize this new chemical, which it called C8. In fact, its existence—and the mounting evidence of its toxicity—was kept a secret from the public for half a century.

In 1961, 3M and DuPont started conducting secret medical studies and amassing reams of evidence that PFOA exposure was linked to several types of cancer, birth defects, and possibly DNA damage. DuPont decided to brush it under the rug and keep raking in the profits.

We know all this because of the work of a corporate environmental lawyer named Rob Bilott, played by Mark Ruffalo in the 2019 film *Dark Waters*. Up until 1999, Bilott had worked to defend chemical companies, negotiating settlements and agreements with the EPA. He didn't see anything wrong with his work—these companies hadn't done anything illegal, or even unusual for the time, when they dumped their waste in rivers or unlined city landfills, and he even saw himself as helping them stay within the current law. But when a West Virginia farmer who knew Bilott's grandmother approached him for help with some dying cows, it set him off on a journey that eventually uncovered DuPont's and 3M's willingness to sacrifice human health at the altar of profit.

Bilott also uncovered just how inadequate the 1976 Toxic Substances Control Act is. We have a close to fifty-year-old law that effectively relies on corporations to police themselves when it comes to toxic chemicals. Our fallback when this fails is to hope that a plucky lawyer gets lucky enough to uncover the secrets of these corporations, and that he can prove, without a doubt, that they knew they were poisoning us.

In May 2000, 3M announced it would phase C8 out. But the fashion industry was already hooked, and DuPont was there to sell this magic stuff to textile mills. Put on textiles, perfluorinated chemicals do a lovely job of repelling both stains and water, while keeping fabric lightweight and breathable. They've ended up seasoning anything and everything that could use a little water-proofing: hiking boots, raincoats, ski and snowboard suits, even bathing suits, so you wouldn't even need a towel to walk from the pool to the hotel bar. Why not? Brands demand performance, and manufacturers are going to give it to them.

This lackadaisical attitude, coupled with the fact that these chemicals never degrade, means they are now everywhere. PFOA has been found in animals in the Antarctic and in the blood of 99.7 percent of Americans. It's in the rainwater falling everywhere on earth.

"While we were trying to get some of the worst PFAS compounds out of the environment, and that's, you know, nearly an impossible task, these things don't break down—companies were adding and using more and more of these newer perfluorinated compounds," Muhannad Malas told me about his time campaigning against toxic chemicals in Canada. "We're now dealing with a class of at least five thousand of them, many of them we don't know about. We just know they exist. We don't know what their actual impacts are. They don't even have names yet. They have not been risk assessed by a regulatory body. And, you know, what you see as a consumer is, oh, these socks are waterproof."

As late as 2011, Twin Hill was telling Alaska Airlines that Teflon, DuPont's perfluorinated coating, was on its uniforms and was perfectly safe. But flight attendants weren't the only professionals concerned about their uniforms.

Paul Cotter, a firefighter from Massachusetts, was diagnosed with cancer in 2014. It ended his career and also raised some unsettling questions. Why did four men in his twelve-man truck have cancer? And why were cancer rates for firefighters rising, becoming their leading cause of death, even as their respiratory protective gear got better? Firefighters have a 14 percent higher risk of dying from cancer—mainly testicular, mesothelioma, and non-Hodgkin's lymphoma—than the general population of the US. Could it be not because of what is in the smoke but because of something on the uniforms themselves? Paul and his wife, Diane, suspected that the perfluorinated coating was the culprit.

Before the turn of the century, a polyurethane barrier kept firefighters dry when entering a building being blasted by hoses. But in the mid-2000s, research funded by DuPont and the uniform maker Lion came out, showing that when polyurethane is put under a xenon lamp for a few hours, it is prone to harden, crack, and fail. Never mind that as a liner, the polyurethane wouldn't even be exposed to sunlight or UV rays, especially the kind in a xenon lamp. But the National Fire Protection Association took the research at face value and started requiring all turnout gear to have a Teflon lining. DuPont and Gore, maker of Gore-Tex, profited handsomely from this policy change. So did Milliken, which also made water-resistant and fireproof textiles.

In 2006, the EPA had "invited" perfluorinated product manufactures to phase out PFOA and PFOS by 2015. No more Scotchgard? Well, not quite. These two chemicals were merely replaced with other cousins, what are called "short-chain" PFAS. Because we believed at the time—mistakenly—that they stay in the human body for a shorter amount of time, they are marketed as safer. But the short-chain PFAS have to be used at higher amounts and are more water soluble, meaning they wash off more readily from treated textiles, and travel farther and faster in waterways. And as short-chain chemicals undergo more scrutiny, they're being linked to similar health outcomes as PFOA exposure. The EPA's latest estimate of the number of types of PFAS in existence is more than twelve thousand.

In an email to a Nantucket firefighter in the summer of 2020, a representative from Milliken repeated twice that "not all PFAS chemicals are bad."

"I suggest that instead of touting the safety of chemicals that have not been adequately studied, you and the rest of the industry get together and offer us an alternative," the firefighter shot back. If only that was how this ever worked.

Confused and getting no support from the firefighters' union, which had a financial arrangement with the uniform makers, the Cotters heard about a professor at Notre Dame who might be able to help them, a Dr. Graham Peaslee.

Intentionally Added

When I first saw Peaslee's name in a story about the toxic "forever chemicals" in everyday household items, I was confused. Why was a nuclear physics professor involved in a textile chemistry fight? But his name kept coming up—first in a Sierra Club investigation into toxic period panties, and then in emails forwarded from a flight attendant. The Association of Flight Attendants' Judith Anderson had shipped him forty-two navy-blue uniform pieces to test.

It was late 2021, I had been researching this topic for months, and so far, I had been able to find almost no independent researchers who knew anything about toxic chemicals in fashion. Most said they didn't know anything about fashion. Or they had done consulting work for the industry and so had signed an NDA or three, and could talk only very carefully and in generalities. They tended to say everything was fine. The brands have it handled.

I was getting desperate for an unbiased view. So I emailed Peaslee, and he quickly responded and agreed to an interview. In his early sixties, Peaslee looks like a scientist, with conservative button-downs and brown-rimmed glasses. He talks fast, as if trying to cram a three-hour seminar into one hour, and is unflappably cheerful, a wry smile dancing on his face even while describing the "nasty things" chemical and fashion industry folks say about him.

His journey down the fashion rabbit hole started around 2013, when the chemist and advocate Arlene Blum gave a presentation at his university on brominated flame retardants. Used on everything from couches to electronics, this extremely toxic class of flame retardants is a notorious endocrine disruptor, and Blum was on a mission to get them banned. Peaslee realized he could quickly measure the level of brominated flame retardants in consumer products using an X-ray technique, and he embarked on a series of research projects with Blum to do just that. His results, cataloged in a series in the *Chicago Tribune*, gave clean chemistry advocates crucial ammunition in the fight to convince state legislatures to ban the use of toxic flame retardants in consumer products.

Then, an expert on perfluorinated chemicals got in touch and asked him if he could do the same for her. Peaslee realized he could use an old nuclear technique, something called particle-induced gamma-ray emission (PIGE, pronounced *piggy*) spectroscopy, that can measure fluorine.

Fluorine by itself is fine. But when you find more than 100 ppm of it on a garment, a reasonable assumption is that it was intentionally added. And the only reason to add fluorine to a garment is to achieve the water and stain repellency that comes from per- and polyfluorinated chemistry.

So he called back the researcher who was asking him if he could measure PFAS on clothing and asked her to send him something with a fluorinated finish. She sent him a pair of Dockers stain-resistant work pants. He put them under the beam, and less than a minute later, he had his answer.

"We discovered we had a technique that nobody else had, that we could measure this stuff in thirty or sixty seconds," he said.

What was even better is that this new technique could measure the presence of *all* fluorinated chemicals. Most tests looked only for a couple dozen of the most commonly used PFAS, which left the door wide open for manufacturers to switch to one of the other thousands of PFAS variations and avoid detection. Now, they had nowhere to hide.

Yes, the PIGE test would come up positive for benign fluorine in things like toothpaste and Prozac, so to be conclusive, it does require further testing for specific types of PFAS. But when it comes to fashion, the most reasonable conclusion is that the high amounts of fluorine are there because of PFAS chemicals.

Peaslee and his students had a fun new toy, and when on a whim they decided to put a burger wrapper from a local fast-food chain under the beam, they made a nasty discovery. That led to an industry-rocking 2017 study that found evidence of PFAS coating cardboard packaging and paper food wrappers collected from fast-food restaurants.

Now Peaslee and his students were testing all sorts of things and finding PFAS. They found it in quick-dry bathing suits. A cop sent them his uniform when he noticed it had a California Prop 65 label saying it contained a known carcinogen. Most important, however, was the fact that Peaslee was doing all this testing for free. It didn't cost him much—maybe twenty dollars per test—and it was good practice for his students. They seemed to find PFAS almost everywhere they looked.

It was around Halloween when the firefighters' uniforms arrived at his lab, and a couple of students tried them on for a costume. "Those are samples. Take them off," Peaslee admonished his students. They did, but first put the lab safety gloves they had been wearing when handling the turnout gear under the beam. The gloves, which had been fluorine-free, now had PFAS on them. This was important because it showed—contrary to the chemical industry's story—that PFAS could slough off fabrics. And if it could do that, it means that we can ingest them.

When Peaslee started testing the turnout gear itself, he found that the PFAS was shedding off the gear at the rate of parts-per-million level. When it accumulates in the blood, it's considered toxic at the parts-per-*billion* level, a thousand times less. Each firefighting uniform contained a pound and a half of the chemical. The firefighters were wearing their turnout gear all the time, even when off duty, getting it all over their skin and breathing in PFAS dust day in and day out. "That's a chronic exposure as opposed to an acute exposure," Peaslee said. "And then all bets are off."

Peaslee was starting to wonder whether PFAS, which has been shown to suppress the immune system, was making firefighters more prone to all types of cancer, not just ones directly linked to PFAS.

So was the government. In 2022, as the EPA hinted that it would classify all PFAS as hazardous, Milliken saw the writing on the wall. It announced that it would phase out the use of PFAS in all its performance fabrics.

But you have to remember, Milliken does much of its manufacturing here, and has stayed within legal boundaries. For factories located abroad in developing countries, outside the reach of the EPA, there's little stopping them from dousing your children's raincoats in a PFAS-based, durable water repellent.

Or, for that matter, as we'll see, putting PFAS in supposedly eco-friendly and certified-safe products.

CHAPTER 4

DANGEROUS DYES

From Venomous Greens to Coal Tar Colors

So much of what historically made fashion dangerous to our health has been invisible. It sheds microscopic dust, mingles with our sweat, or wafts off with just a whiff of chemical smell, if it has any odor at all. Without the help of expensive testing equipment, we would never know that it's there.

The most toxic product of the Industrial Revolution, however, has been right in front of our eyes all along. Yet somehow, when it comes to the bright colors created out of some of the most ubiquitous carcinogenic substances known to modern man, we've had the wool pulled over our eyes.

Venomous Greens

On a November morning in 1861, according to Matthews David in her book *Fashion Victims: The Dangers of Dress Past and Present,* a young London woman picked her way through the city's dirty streets to the artificial flower atelier where she worked. Nineteen-year-old Matilda Scheurer was probably a pathetic sight, with bloodied bandages wrapped around the open sores on her hands.

Her green-rimmed fingernails, with skin peeling away from the nail beds, were left exposed to the sooty air. The skin around her nostrils would have been red, peeling, and chapped. If there was a latrine near the workshop, she might have rushed to it upon arrival, because of her diarrhea. Her head likely felt as though it was being squeezed in a vise. Her condition, to quote a contemporary doctor, was "wretched in the extreme."

Her job was to dust green pigment onto fake leaves, which would then be shaped into exquisite floral crowns. Adorned with delicate flowers, twisted vines, plump strawberries and grapes, and lush leaves, these headpieces looked as though they had been plucked and arranged by a nymph . . . or a servant at a country estate.

Matilda had fallen ill four times in the previous eighteen months, and her mother later told the press that her other daughter, who also worked making faux flowers, had already passed away. Matilda probably knew she was not long for this world. As one of her compatriots sobbed, according to the *English Woman's Journal* in 1861, "I saw the ladies had all handkerchiefs on their faces and some of 'em was soaked in blood, and some of their ears is almost dropping off. I won't do 'em. If I am to be poisoned, I'll be poisoned at once. Not by inches."

But what choice did she have? Like generations of young, poor women around the world, crafting confections for the consumer class was her only way to make money.

In 1778, the famous German chemist Carl Wilhelm Scheele released his recipe for the first green pigment, a combination of arsenic trioxide, or white arsenic, and copper. This was an electrifying development. Before this point, dyeing anything green was exceedingly difficult and expensive, involving layering fickle yellow dyes on top of even more fickle indigo-blue dyes. Green was a color reserved for the kind of people who owned their own countryside estates.

As Romanticism, which emphasized the natural and green, swept through the salons of Europe, Scheele's green, as it was known, became wildly popular for use in everything from candies and children's toys to candles and especially wallpaper. When copper acetoarsenite, a more brilliant and saturated pigment, was synthesized in 1814, green took the fashion world by storm. As the Victorian age dawned in England, the most stylish ladies swathed themselves in emerald-green dresses and Paris-green shawls. Little girls wore *beau vert* dresses. And what was prized more than anything were green-hued leaves and flowers that adorned the most fashionable heads, hats, and frocks across the European continent.

By 1858, there were more than eighteen thousand faux flower makers between Paris and Great Britain, most of them staffed by young women working in appalling conditions. In 1859, a high-ranking French physician (perhaps one of the first industrial hygienists and an early forebear to Judith Anderson at the Association of Flight Attendants) named Ange-Gabriel-Maxime Vernois published an illustrated book with detailed chromolithograph illustrations showing open sores on the hands and legs of flower makers, and their red, raw nostrils.

While the public was well aware of arsenic's use as a sneaky murder weapon, everyone—including the government—had a lax attitude toward it in everyday life. A fine white powder that was odorless and colorless, arsenic was such a cheap and common household substance that, upon seeing a rat sniffing around the larder, a mother could send a child to the pharmacy to fetch her some with nary a raised eyebrow. France finally banned the pigment from commercial use in 1846, but Britain's Sale of Arsenic Regulation Act of 1851 and the Pharmacy Act of 1868 in Britain only limited the amount that could be sold to individual consumers. Dyehouses continued to have unfettered access.

It took an "accidental" death to catch the city's attention. That day in November, when flower maker Matilda Scheurer finally succumbed to Paris green's caustic effects, it was a long and painful death. When the doctor arrived, she was vomiting green bile and begging for water, looking through eyes that saw only green. Her final hours were spent in convulsions; she was foaming from her mouth, eyes, and nose.

An inquest was held to determine fault, but the jury decided that it was an accident "occasioned by arsenite of copper used in her employment." This passive voice did not fool observers. A writer for the British satirical magazine *Punch* wrote, "Death is evidently about as accidental as it is when resulting from a railway collision occasioned by arrangements known to be faulty."

But instead of blaming the (male) workshop owner or the (male-owned) dye manufacturers who had profited off Matilda's slow poisoning, the lettered men of the era laid the blame at the silk-slippered feet of the ladies who bought the flower crowns. The *Punch* author urged its male readers to shame any female dance partner who happened to be wearing a green headdress. "Treat the practice of poisoning the artificial flowers-makers with sufficient levity, not censuring it in strong or serious language, but only saying, for instance, that you think it jolly avaricious, and delightfully inhuman," the author sneered. "Girls in these green dresses ought to be marked 'DANGEROUS!' or to have 'BEWARE OF POISON!' embroidered in red letters right across their backs," another *Punch* article said.

(This attitude continues today on a grand scale, as microinfluencers are shamed on social media for tagging fast-fashion brands, while the male founders of those brands avoid media attention—even though they consistently rank in the top twenty of the world's richest billionaires.)

Some ladies of the late 1800s took the criticism to heart, and they in turn launched what might have been the first ethical fashion campaign. When the Ladies' Sanitary Association asked a professor at the London College of Chemistry to test the green leaves in a typical headdress, he found it contained enough arsenic to kill up to twenty people.

In June 1862, the *English Woman's Journal* again entreated its readers to move on from green. They quoted a physician who said,

"Emerald green is exceedingly injurious to the wearer. Head-ache, and sometimes erysipelas [an infection of the skin] is the unsuspected result of green wreaths." The writer shared anecdotes of wreath wearers losing hair and their foreheads erupting in a rash.

A Berlin doctor estimated that a typical green ball gown would shed enough arsenic powder in an evening to kill twelve. "The colouring matter is loosely held on with starch, and as the wearer is whirled along in the waltz she throws off a cloud of poisoned dust, which tells its tale in the parched throat and swollen eyelids of the next morning," the *Medical Times and Gazette* wrote in February 1862.

After a teenager died from sucking the paint off an arsenical green grape, Victorians flew into full arsenic terror. According to Simon Garfield's 2000 book *Mauve: How One Man Invented a Colour That Changed the World*, arsenic green had been banned in Bavaria by 1862. But a committee of chemists, dyers, and doctors that was convened by the Royal Society of Arts to consider the problem concluded that the answer was simply to educate the public on the dangers of buying green wallpaper. The public was officially left to fend for themselves against arsenic fashion's ravages, as if it were a disease or God's will, and not a man-made substance filling the coffers of the business elite.

As new synthetic green dyes came to market in the 1870s, fashion houses began to claim that their green wares were *not* made with arsenic. But of course, that wasn't always true. In 1871, *Medical Press and Circular* reported on a lady who suffered skin ulcerations around her fingernails, until she realized the culprit was her new green gloves, bought from a "respectable" fashion house. (Catherine de' Medici might have felt vindicated with this proof that arsenic gloves would take years, not days, to kill their wearer.)

In fact, arsenic could be found now in a whole range of colors, since using arsenic acid with the new synthetic dyes tended to make them brighter. In 1863, people living near a synthetic dye factory of J. J. Muller-Pack and Co. in Basel, Switzerland, began to fall ill after drinking water from their wells. A chemist determined that the arsenic levels were "so high the water must be designated as poisoned." Muller-Pack and Co. was found guilty of gross negligence, fined, and forced to compensate the victims and nearby landowners. (It is possible, as we will see, that it was more than just arsenic that caused the "indefinable, peculiar, and somewhat repulsive odor" in the water.)

German dye companies were not so easily cowed. In 1870, concerned about reports of skin inflammation caused by dyed women's fashion accessories, the German government sponsored a study on the issue. One Dr. Springmuhl tested fourteen samples of dye and found that nine of them contained at least 2 percent arsenic. Five of them contained more than 4.3 percent. He also found after the wool had been washed just once, substantial traces of arsenic had ended up in the water. This suggested, at least for some of the cheaper dyes, that sweating in arsenic green or other dyed clothing could be dangerous, and that the arsenic was likely finding its way into the local water sources.

That was not the result Germany's economically powerful dye industry wanted to hear. The German government, acquiescing to the dyers' demands, announced that women had nothing to fear from synthetically dyed fashion. But by the end of the century, arsenic use in fashion was becoming untenable and falling out of use. Though, as in many of these cases, it was never completely banished.

Brighter Living Through Chemistry

It was an exciting time to be a chemist in the early 1800s. It was a new field, only recently separated from physics, and scientists were busy theorizing and discovering all the laws that governed chemical reactions. They didn't fully understand what was happening in their beakers, but they were starting to name and categorize elements and compounds, and finding that if they heated these compounds and threw them together in a beaker, they could produce wondrous new colors and substances—if they didn't get their faces burned off by an explosion first. An English scientist discovered the chemical benzene in 1825. A Prussian chemist discovered liquid aniline the next year. In 1832, a German chemist took benzene and synthesized nitrobenzene.

Scientists understood even less about the impact of these substances on human health. That would come much later, after this Pandora's box of compounds had been unleashed on the public. Benzene can cause leukemia. Acute aniline poisoning can be fatal, and long-term exposure is suspected to cause cancer, at least in rats. Nitrobenzene would end up acting as fashion's first real contact poison—meaning just having it on your skin can lead to poisoning and death. These chemists had been working with plant-based components in their experiments, but plant-based ingredients were limited, unreliable, and expensive to procure. It would be much easier and cheaper to use something that companies would literally give away. Coal tar, the waste product of making coal gas and coke (not the illegal drug or the beverage but a fuel product derived from burning coal at high temperatures), was exactly that: a massively overabundant, noxious waste sludge produced by the Industrial Revolution.

So the founding director of England's Royal College of Chemistry, a German chemist by the name of August Wilhelm von Hofmann, set to work isolating coal tar's various components. His first chemical product from coal tar was benzene in 1845. Within two years, a British chemist had patented nitrobenzene from coal tar and was selling it to perfumeries.

Hofmann wanted to figure out what to do with a class of compounds called amines, many of which later turned out to be carcinogenic. In 1856, he tasked a precocious eighteen-year-old British student of his, William Perkin, with trying to synthesize quinine out of coal tar to help combat malaria.

When Perkin mixed aniline derived from benzene with potassium dichromate and sulfuric acid, a black substance precipitated out of the solution to the bottom of the test tube. When he tried dipping a rag in alcohol to clean the tube, he found himself with a piece of gorgeous purple fabric.

Up to that point, fashion's palette was rather dull. With enough skill and resources, a dyer could achieve shades of yellow, blue, and purple using plants and flowers. When Spain colonized what is now Mexico, they started shipping back logwood, which made black, purple, and gray, and a tiny cactus pest called the cochineal bug, which provided dyers with brilliant red, orange, and purple. And of course, the bright green, arsenic-derived hues were well established. But for the most part, the regular person's dress in Europe was limited to muted shades of yellow, gray, and brown, and most colors tended to fade in the wash.

As Simon Garfield explained in *Mauve*, a history of Perkin and his invention, chemists often tossed out beakers with colored compounds, not realizing their immense commercial possibilities. "In the unlikely event that a scientist would have thought a particular tint might be useful in the dyeing of a woman's dress, they would most certainly have believed such fripperies unworthy of their calling," Garfield wrote.

This day was different. When Perkin showed the dyed cloth to friends, they encouraged him to try to manufacture it on a large scale. After all, many men were making their fortunes in the rapidly expanding textile industry. Perkin convinced his father and brother to go in with him on the venture.

They looked for a good site in London for their factory but were stymied by local planning authorities who, thanks to newspaper reports, were already aware of the offensive air and water pollution flowing from newfangled chemical manufacturing plants.

Finally, the Perkin men secured a spot northwest of London and built a factory over the next six months. While that was happening, Perkin set up a workshop nearby to continue experimentation. "Poor ventilation meant he frequently abandoned his work when overcome with vapors," Garfield wrote.

Aniline was in short supply, so Perkin designed and installed machines that could produce it from nitrobenzene, the early versions of which were highly combustible. An editor wrote a century later in the trade journal *International Dyer, Textile Printer, Bleacher and Finisher*, "In those early, groping stages of manufacture it is a miracle that Perkin did not blow himself and Greenford Green"—the hamlet where he situated his factory—"to pieces."

Mad for Magenta

When you look at John Phillip's painting *The Marriage of Victoria, Princess Royal*, your eye is immediately drawn to Queen Victoria standing on the right. Her gown, with its deep V-neck, puffed short sleeves, and large, hooped skirt, is made of arresting lilac velvet that fairly glows against the pale pastels of the other court ladies. To achieve such a saturated color, the dyehouse supplying Victoria's designer likely would have painstakingly dyed the silk using various lichens. If the royal laundry had attempted to wash it, it would have been ruined. It was a dress that hardly anyone but the aristocracy could afford to wear.

Luckily, that was the exact color coming out of Perkin's factory. By the middle of 1859, Perkin was shipping out "vast quantities" of what he called "mauvine" to eager dyehouses in Britain. "They were clamorous for it," Perkin later said. French dyehouses in Lyon had figured out how to make it on their own by getting copies of scientific speeches on the subject. *Mauve*—the French word for the flower mallow—was everywhere: on feathered fans, striped gowns, gloves, and ribbons. *Punch* warned in 1859 of a plague of "mauve measles" and suggested that hat shops be marked as "Dangerous." It was a joke, but the magazine's analogy for mauve's viral spread through the populace was perhaps more apt than they knew.

The mauve craze was a purple flash in the pan. Within a couple of years, it was replaced by fuchsia, a saturated purple-red, then Hofmann's violet. A Cambrian explosion of dye ensued: scarlet from anthracene (which we now know can cause skin allergies), pink from phenol (kidney damage, skin burns, convulsions), magenta from toluene (birth defects and pregnancy loss, liver damage, central nervous system damage). The Grand Junction Canal outside the Perkin & Sons factory turned a different color every week.

It was as if the erstwhile muted world of fashion had been swept up in a tornado and set back down in the Land of Oz. And everyone—royals, middle-class women, and even their servants—were all welcome to walk this multicolor road into the future. Magazines aimed at middle-class women in Britain and America, with headlines like "Colour in the Coal-Scuttle," encouraged them to learn about chemistry and the new topic of color theory so they could better dress their households when presented with an infinite array of colors, instead of just easily matched earth tones.

In 1884, the first direct dye—that is, a dye that doesn't require a chemical called a mordant to fix it to the fabric—was marketed by a German dye company. Made using the chemical benzidine, which was later connected to bladder cancer in dye factory workers, it was named Congo red. (Bloody and violent colonization was a trendy topic among industrialists at the time.)

Synthetic indigo hit the market in 1897 and quickly decimated the British-controlled Indian indigo industry. Though wealthy British planters disliked this turn of events, the workers who labored in the indigo fields and waded around in vats of fermenting indigo were happy to see the industry go. Later, an independent

India and China would wrest control of dye production, and its pollution, back from the British. But only after it had ceased to be an exciting and profitable technology.

In 1873, at age thirty-five, Perkin got out of the business. Two bad accidents at his factory the prior year weighed on his conscience, and he couldn't compete against the German and Swiss companies that had popped up. Some of them—Bayer, BASF, Ciba, and Geigy (the latter two eventually merged and became Novartis)—are still operating today, albeit as chemical and pharmaceutical companies.

In 1875, BASF started manufacturing azo dyes, that class of dyes that so bedeviled our intrepid Duke researchers in chapter 2. By the end of the century, chemists had left behind coal sludge waste and were transforming petroleum into valuable chemicals and materials.

It wasn't long before reports started surfacing in the *Times* (UK) of bright red, orange, and fuchsia socks that were causing pain, swelling, skin eruptions, and even lameness in consumers. A British member of Parliament was confined to his house for months to allow his feet to heal. A Frenchman in Le Havre, after wearing his new striped socks for twelve days, found his feet had stripes of eczema and pustules. The public started to panic, and one respected fashion house in Britain decided to stop their order of six thousand pairs of tainted socks and return to traditional dyes.

In 1869, according to Matthews David, two French toxicologists decided to do an experiment. They boiled socks in alcohol and injected the distilled coralline color, a popular shade of red, into a dog, rabbit, and frog. All three died. Just to drive the point home, they then took the red-stained lungs of the rabbit, extracted the dye, and used it to dye a skein of silk red again.

Lyon's dye industry was not amused and, in response, enlisted the help of two Lyonnaise brothers, a doctor and a veterinarian. They used alcohol to distill the dye out of colorful socks and proceeded to dye their own hands and feet many times to prove it was completely safe. (There is always someone willing to accept money in exchange for calming the public's fears.)

Doctors were puzzled. Why did some people react so strongly to aniline-dyed socks, while others were just fine? A judge in a poisonous sock case brought up the fact that he himself enjoyed colorful socks without suffering chemical burns. Thus began a long tradition of authority figures downplaying the experience of the portion of people who have acute, painful reactions to dyes and finishes. Even though, in many cases, the skin reactions of the few were the body sending up flares for help, before things got deadly.

But there were at least two scientists who believed people when they said toxic dyes were making them sick: Gustav Jäger in Germany and James Startin in England.

James Startin's exhibit at the 1884 International Health Exhibition caused a sensation. The surgeon and lecturer at St. John's Hospital for Diseases of the Skin in London had received so many visits from patients suffering from painful rashes from aniline-dyed stockings and gloves that he started taking pictures. He hung them at the exhibition for the benefit of wide-eyed crowds.

The dye industry first tried to wine and dine Startin over to their side. When that didn't work, they set out to malign his work. "We want the truth, and well authenticated cases, and proof that aniline dye has produced the injurious effect alleged," a member of the Society of Dyers and Colourists sniffed. "Fortunately, chemistry is a science which deals only with facts. It does not deal with speculative opinions or sensational exhibits."

But at least another man of science and facts felt stymied by the dye industry's secrecy. "The difficulties which surround the investigation of this subject, whether from a scientific or a practical point of view, are considerable," wrote German physician Gustav Jäger. "In the first place, many different chemical substances and combinations of substances have to be taken into account; secondly, the matter is embarrassed by the difficulty of ascertaining with what dye a material has been treated . . . the material may have passed through several hands after it has left the dyer, who, moreover, often regards his method of procedure as a business secret."

These are many of the same complaints I heard from researchers in 2022.

Jäger was a kind of Renaissance man of science. Born in 1832 in a small town in southwestern Germany and educated at a German medical school, he devised scientific theories that were the rough precursors to fields of study we now know as pheromones and genetics. Pictures of him across the decades show a sturdy, serious man with dark hair, a beard, and an impressive waxed handlebar mustache. He is always wearing some version of a fitted wool suit.

Jäger was deeply concerned about aniline dyes. "The assertion that aniline dyes are only injurious when they contain arsenic, is entirely erroneous; they are chiefly noxious because of their volatility," he wrote. In other words, they can easily come off the fabric as fumes or in sweat. In 1880, he published the first of several booklets on the topic of healthy fashion, *Standardized Apparel for Health Protection*. In it, he distilled his theories to this basic advice: wear only undyed animal fibers, especially wool, next to the skin.

Thanks to Jäger and Startin, consumers who were educated enough to understand aniline's perils now boasted of buying artisanal, vegetable-dyed stockings made by country peasants. The upper classes were seized with "chromophobia"—bright colors were now regarded as tacky. As germ theory took hold, pure white dresses that could be bleached and washed in scalding hot water came into vogue.

A British entrepreneur licensed Dr. Jäger's name and launched a range of performance clothing and undergarments called Jaeger's Sanitary Woollens—the first consumer clothing line marketed to consumers as natural and nontoxic. "Because it is made from carefully selected natural (undyed) wool, this wool is far more durable than wool which has been dyed and chemically treated," promised a 1907 Jaeger print advertisement with an illustration of a woman in a smart, bustled dress. You can still see one of Jaeger's finely woven wool corsets from the 1890s at the Fashion Institute of Design and Merchandising Museum in Los Angeles. It looks like the coziest corset ever made, and presaged pediatric nurse Karly Hiser's homemade underwear for her son by 130 years.

Over the course of its 133-year run, Jaeger counted among its fans explorer Ernest Shackleton, Audrey Hepburn, and Marilyn Monroe. Unfortunately, the brand fell out of favor in the latter half of the twentieth century and went into administration—that's British for bankruptcy—in 2017. Jäger would have been pleased as punch to see merino wool's recent comeback in everything from sneakers to T-shirts. It's marketed as a natural, sweat-wicking, anti-odor alternative to synthetic fibers. He would probably be less pleased to learn what kind of toxic chemicals were found on wool garments in 2021.

Black Death

It wasn't just bright-hued fabric dyes that caused problems. Starting around the mid-1800s, upon the death of a loved one, European and American women of all classes were expected to don elaborate mourning fashion made with mourning crape, a matte black silk. Made from waste silk that was dyed black, crimped, and stiffened with glue, gum, or starch, it was cheap to make and enormously profitable. In 1865, the leading mourning crape manufacturer, the British company Courtaulds, garnered a 30 percent profit margin on $127,000 in revenue in one year alone, the equivalent of over $2 million today.

But for women, it was thick, cumbersome, and on the whole

very unpleasant. When black crape got wet, the dye ran and stained the wearer's skin. Women were told to use a rather poisonous mix of oxalic acid and cream of tartar to rub it off.

By the 1880s, even the most proper women were fed up with it. It was "most unhealthy: it harms the eyes and it injures the skin," the etiquette expert Mrs. John Sherwood wrote in 1884. The medical community agreed. "I have frequently been consulted for an eczemaform eruption of the face occasioned by wearing mourning veils of *crèpe*," Dr. Prince A. Morrow wrote in an 1894 book on dermatology. Both the *New York Medical Journal* and the *Northwestern Lancet* said the "poisonous" and "toxic" particles that floated off the crape as it rubbed against itself and the skin were causing respiratory illnesses. "Many a woman has been laid in her coffin by the wearing of crape," declared the doctor in his letter to the editor.

Whether or not that was hyperbole, women had had enough. Between 1883 and 1894, Courtaulds' sales plummeted 62 percent, and it was forced to turn to selling silks in other colors.

But black is always in style. And nitrobenzene, used as a solvent in liquid blacking solution for shoes, was by far the worst dye chemical of all. When inhaled or absorbed through the skin in high enough doses, it impairs the body's ability to deliver fresh oxygen to tissue, a condition now known as methemoglobinemia. This manifests as dizziness and fatigue, blue lips and skin, and eventually death. It was especially dangerous for those who used it on cloth shoes, were too impatient to wait for it to dry, and exerted themselves dancing or walking in hot weather.

In 1900, a French family was planning an outing to the beach with their seven children. At the time, days at the beach were a proper social occasion, which called for appropriate footwear. So the family used shoe blacking to make their children's shoes look new. Once they got to the beach, the children must have gotten sweaty running and playing in the hot sand.

Poison, as a rule, affects the littlest bodies the most, and the most swiftly. First, the three-year-old daughter's lips turned blue. Moments after she passed out, the four-year-old exclaimed, "*Maman*, everything is spinning!" before falling to the ground. The five-year-old brother followed a half hour later. The parents saw the lips and hands of their children ages nine, thirteen, and fourteen also turn blue, though they managed to stay conscious.

The report on this terrifying incident was published by a pair of French doctors, Louis Landouzy and Paul Brouardel, who were also involved in another French court case against a manufacturer of toxic shoe dye. In this case, a Sieur W. blacked his shoes the night before walking three kilometers across Paris to his job. By midmorning, Sieur W. felt dizzy and his lips and face had turned a frightening shade of violet. When he made it to the hospital and took off his "accursed" dyed boots, he started to recover.

Landouzy and Brouardel, as expert witnesses, demonstrated to the court the potency of the poisonous shoe dye on a doomed rabbit. They shaved its hair, applied a strip of leather dyed with the shoe blacking, and over that applied a band of cotton wet with hot water to mimic the effect of sweaty feet in socks. Within two hours, the rabbit had turned blue and died. The court condemned the manufacturer and slapped him with a fifty-franc fine, or the equivalent of less than two hundred euros today.

"It is essential to warn the public that aniline dyes and shoe polish are dangerous products," a medical student in Lyon wrote in 1901 for his thesis. He advocated for clear labels and regulation of toxic shoe blacking. Even though this stuff had been in circulation for decades, it would be several more decades before any government would oblige.

In March 1904, four years after the incident on the French beach, a healthy twenty-two-year-old salesman in Toledo, Ohio, died after painting the canvas tops of his new shoes with shoe blacking and going out dancing with friends. Two decades later, four students at the University of Michigan were poisoned. They all survived, but one required two blood transfusions, according to Matthews David.

A government finally swung into action. In 1927, the Department of Health in Chicago banned all leather dyes containing toxic solvents and required warning labels on shoe blacking, instructing consumers to use it only on leather, not canvas, and to wait seventy-two hours before putting on blacked shoes. Warning signs were placed in shoe stores, shoe repair shops, and shoeshine parlors—though illiterate or immigrant shoe shiners might not have been able to read these warnings.

It wasn't just shoes, however, that could use a little blacking. In the early twentieth century, the German chemical industry introduced a synthetic dye named Ursol to the American market, to be used for both furs and women's hair and eyelashes. Some furriers used it to transform cheap furs like rabbit and goat into fake sable and black bear, and were rewarded with eczema, breathing and intestinal problems, and inflammation of the eyes. The cheap fur also caused some nasty cases of contact dermatitis in their customers.

One woman who had her eyelashes dyed black in 1933 had such a terrible reaction that she ended up losing her vision. Her daughter, Hazel Fay Musser, wrote a letter to President Franklin D. Roosevelt, helping the administration sign into place the Food, Drug, and Cosmetic Act of 1938.

The new legislation did not include clothing.

Beyond an Unreasonable Doubt

If some consumers were suffering skin and respiratory reactions to nitrobenzene, the scene in the dye factories was worse. A worker died after having his clothes splashed with nitrobenzene. Dyehouse workers who came in contact with aniline dye developed a condition called anilinism, in which the red blood cells are destroyed, causing anemia, headaches, tremor, pain and a burning sensation in the hands and feet, cardiac arrhythmia, and eventually narcosis or coma. (This isn't a relic of the past. Over Christmas supper in Mississippi, a distant relative, a soft-spoken, lanky man with a thick drawl, told me about his time working at the First Chemical aniline plant in Pascagoula. He has taken coworkers suffering from anilinism to the nearby hospital several times.)

In 1895, German surgeon Ludwig W. C. Rehn reported that three of the forty-five workers in a factory producing the trendy color fuchsia had developed bladder cancer, and many more developed malignant bladder disease. When more bladder cancer clusters appeared in Basel and elsewhere in Germany, Swiss and German scientists conceded at a 1913 conference that something in the aniline dye factories was causing the outbreaks.

The First World War prompted Germany's chemical factories to pivot to explosives, and by 1919, eighty factories in the US were busily producing aniline dyes, including the new chemical company DuPont. Over the next century, DuPont—the same chemical company that dumped toxic PFAS into the water in West Virginia—would develop a reputation first as a leading producer of innovative materials and chemicals, and then as a brazen producer of poisons.

In 1921, the International Labor Office confirmed that it was the ingredients benzidine and beta-naphthylamine (BNA) causing bladder cancer in dye factory workers, and in 1932, DuPont physicians identified its own first cases at its New Jersey factory. At first, DuPont was open to studying the issue, and even funded research on the topic. But after this brief period of scientific inquiry, DuPont forbade its lead pathologist from publishing his research and fired him. DuPont did not upgrade its BNA factory to protect its workers until 1951, "more than 35 years after BNA production began and 20 years after it knew the epidemic was recognized," David Michaels wrote in his damning 1988 report, "Waiting for the Body Count: Corporate Decision Making and Bladder Cancer in the U.S. Dye Industry." As the years passed, identical stories played out at other aniline dye plants in the US and abroad: discover some cases of cancer, ask someone reputable to study it, bury the evidence, keep producing the dye as before and polluting both the workers and the surrounding community.

In his 1988 report, Michaels counted seven documented outbreaks and at least 750 individual cases of occupational bladder cancer since the 1930s. The Eastern Seaboard of the United States is littered with toxic sites related to shuttered fabric mills and dye factories, and the federal government has spent millions trying to clean these sites up. "It is unrealistic to hope that industry will voluntarily protect workers from substances only suspected to be human carcinogens," he wrote. And that was for their own employees. What about people who purchase their products?

In the 1970s, the federal government finally intervened with the Toxic Substances Control Act, which gave the EPA the power to regulate and control toxic chemicals. The only problem was, the EPA permitted almost all the chemicals already in production, some sixty-four thousand of them. And it regards chemicals as innocent until proven guilty. You need multiple studies, which often stretch into decades, to prove beyond a shadow of a doubt that a particular substance causes harm to humans. By that point, it's often too late—the chemicals are out in the world, in our products, in our water, in our bodies.

And that brings us to where we are now, with the chemical industry busily producing secretive azo dyes abroad, as researchers try to prove to this standard that they are toxic to people who wear synthetic fabrics. Many fashion brands and manufacturers started voluntarily phasing some azo dyes out. But there is no global mechanism to enforce this move. And global enforcement is what you would need, since dyes are no longer manufactured in the US. That's a job for India, China, and other countries with low labor costs and lax, if any, regulation.

Today, thanks to synthetic mauve dye, fossil fuels are the basis for an infinite catalog of textile finishes, pesticides, detergents, pharmaceuticals, glues, plastics, faux leathers, synthetic fabrics, inks, and more. Who would have guessed that 150 years after Perkin peered at his purple fabric, chemistry's core role in fashion would be almost entirely and deliberately obscured from consumers? That the average person, when you tell them that each sweater or pair of jeans, socks, or underwear they buy has dozens of different invisible man-made petrochemicals resting quietly on its surface, is incredulous and confused? Chemistry? From fossil fuels? On this cotton T-shirt? Can't be!

It can. Fossil-fuel chemistry is not only used *in* fashion, but as we've seen, it owes its existence to fashion. Chemistry *is* fashion. Fashion is chemistry. But their shared heritage has been locked away like a shameful family secret.

No wonder—there are some skeletons in that closet.

PART III

THE PRICE OF
TOXIC FASHION

CHAPTER 5

DISRUPTING OUR FERTILITY

Endocrine Disruptors and Their Effects on Our Bodies

Candice woke up in the chair at the fertility clinic. She was miserable, the pain of cramps rolling deep through her uterus. But the doctor had good news. He told her they had retrieved fourteen eggs—a pretty good number. Her husband drove her the two hours to their home in rural Texas. There she waited, her hopes and fears gnawing at her. The next morning, she got the call. Ten of the eggs were mature, and two had fertilized. Her heart sank. They had spent $18,000 that they didn't have on this process, $9,000 per egg.

But she forged ahead, still full of hope. She started the progesterone shots the next day, digging a large-gauge needle full of viscous liquid into her hip and then massaging it in. The hormones really threw her for a loop, sending her emotions bouncing in all directions—not that they needed any encouragement.

Another two-hour drive back to the clinic, the gorgeous Texas landscape rolling by. She then watched on the sonogram screen as the two tiny eggs journeyed through the tube and landed in her womb. She hoped they would stay, and grow.

Two days later, they were back at the clinic for a blood test. The news was devastating. The eggs had not implanted. What was more, the doctor informed her, she had poor egg quality. Even if they tried again, spending thousands of dollars more, the chances were low that she'd get the child she so desperately wanted.

"What can I do to improve it?" she asked the doctor.

"There's not much you can do," he said.

It was 2015, and Candice was thirty. She had been trying for four years to get pregnant. She wasn't about to give up now.

"I started researching, researching, researching and I found the book *It Starts with the Egg*. That is the book that changed the trajectory of my life. I read it and a light came on inside me. And then I reread it and then I highlighted it."

In the book, author Rebecca Fett shares that women are born with all their eggs, but in the three to four months before ovulation, you can impact them, either positively or negatively.

The way to do that? Diet and detoxification. "Thankfully, my husband was on board because he wanted a baby, too," Candice said. So she set about turning their lives completely upside down.

Cleaning Up for Baby

Candice's story is becoming increasingly common. In 2020, the market for assisted reproduction was estimated to be $2.3 billion and growing. Women seeking fertility treatment in the US who have a diminished ovarian reserve—a low number of eggs to give in IVF—increased 37 percent from 2004 to 2011. Miscarriage rates in women are also increasing by about 1 percent a year, and it's not because we're waiting longer to start families—the most dramatic fertility reductions are in younger women.

The thing is, nature has been waving red flags for more than thirty years. In the famous Wingspread Statement of 1991, scientists listed all the fertility problems they were noticing in diverse populations of wildlife. Mammals and birds both had low fertility and compromised immune systems. Birds and fish had thyroid dysfunction, their eggs weren't hatching, and when they did have babies, they were born with gross deformities. Scientists warned that unless we got synthetic hormone-disrupting chemicals under control, these problems would become the norm, in both animals and humans. Nothing was done.

But twenty-six years later, in 2017, the world sat up and paid attention when Shanna H. Swan, PhD, published her paper. It was as if a bomb went off, its blast punching out of stuffy conference rooms and university labs and into the public sphere, sparking a worldwide panic. "Temporal Trends in Sperm Count: A Systematic Review and Meta-Regression Analysis" was not pithily named, but its core message was clear: sperm counts have plummeted by more than 50 percent in the previous forty years, and 41 percent of men could be infertile by 2050. (The data is mainly from Western countries that have reliable, long-term data, but there are indications that the same trends are happening in developing countries.)

According to Swan's book, *Count Down: How Our Modern World Is Threatening Sperm Counts, Altering Male and Female Reproductive Development, and Imperiling the Future of the Human Race*, there is a litany of troublesome signs. A study published in 2016 on prospective Boston sperm donors showed that—despite the fact that men were on average exercising more and drinking and smoking less—their average sperm concentration, mobility, and count had declined in number and fitness in the ten years from 2003 to 2013. Another study of Chinese sperm donors found the same thing.

Swan put the blame squarely on "the ubiquity of insidiously harmful chemicals in the modern world" and especially "chemicals that interfere with our body's natural hormones." These are endocrine-disrupting chemicals. And they include a lot of fashion's favorite finishes and ingredients: lead, mercury, arsenic, phthalates, APEOs, PFAS, and bisphenol A (BPA) and its cousins BPS and

BPF. There are more than a dozen different types of phthalates alone, and the majority of them are used to make the PVC soft for your shower curtains, pleather skirts, and clear shoe straps.

Endocrine disruptors are especially insidious for a few reasons. One is that your endocrine system isn't just about your sex drive or fertility. As anyone with a thyroid disease can tell you, the endocrine system regulates all the important systems in your body, including your immune system, your brain, your metabolism, and your cardiovascular system. It governs weight management and your energy levels, not to mention your skin's appearance and your ability to fend off illness.

The second scary thing about endocrine disruptors is that they don't follow the old adage "The dose makes the poison." Traditional toxicology has always assumed that the smaller the dose, the less the harm. It follows that scientists can always find an amount below which there's no harm at all. This concept is the premise behind textile limits like Oeko-Tex's that say, for example, that anything below .05 ppm is okay when it comes to total phthalates.

During the course of my research, several men in the fashion-chemistry industry (side note: the textile-chemistry professional club is an overwhelmingly male one) patronizingly told me that even salt and water are toxic at high enough amounts. Which is true . . . for salt and water and formaldehyde.

"I do hope you get the balance right," the CEO of a dye company told me on LinkedIn. "Apple seeds contain arsenic but to get arsenic poisoning you need to eat between 250 and a few thousand apples a day! (In other words it ain't going to happen)."

Setting aside that it's *cyanide* that can come from apple seeds, not arsenic, and also the fact that people aren't unknowingly ingesting apple seeds every day (though there have been some instances of children getting cyanide poisoning from eating apple seeds), this CEO's comment betrays an ignorance of endocrine disruptors, which are way more chaotic than your typical poison or carcinogen. In fact, an emerging theory is that they follow a dose-poison

U curve: chaotic effects at high doses, more subtle effects at middling doses, and unpredictable, cascading effects again at tiny doses. More and more researchers agree that there is no "safe" dose of endocrine disruptors. And yet, we're ingesting them in high amounts. A July 2022 study out of Denmark found that the combined amount of twenty-nine reprotoxic chemicals in men's urine samples far exceeded the current safety threshold, sometimes by as much as a hundred times. The average was seventeen times more toxic than is considered safe for men's semen health.

The Chemical/Fertility Connection

Recently an acquaintance told me she was considering shopping at ultra-fast-fashion brands during her pregnancy—she didn't want to overspend on stuff that she would wear for only a few months. I warned her off it (and told her to try to find some hand-me-downs if she was on a tight budget).

Just reckon with the fact that an amount of an endocrine-disrupting chemical so small as to be equal to a drop in an Olympic-size swimming pool can cross the placenta and measurably affect an embryo, and those changes can be permanent. The doses we are talking about, at parts per *billion*, are absolutely the kinds you can get from wearing fashion containing these substances. For example, Dr. Graham Peaslee's research shows that PFAS comes off of treated textiles at the parts-per-*million* level. That's one thousand times more.

There's evidence that damage caused by endocrine disruptors can be passed from mothers and fathers to children, increasing their risk of developing reproductive abnormalities. The effect of phthalate exposure in pregnant animals and humans on their male babies' genitals has even been given a name: phthalate syndrome. It's especially serious when exposure happens between weeks eight and twelve of pregnancy in women.

According to a 2022 study, when researchers sampled the urine of 171 diverse women across the US (including Puerto Rico), they found 103 chemicals representing nine chemical groups: bactericides, benzophenones, bisphenols (such as BPA), fungicides and herbicides, insecticides, parabens, phthalates and alternative plasticizers (like DINCH), and polycyclic aromatic hydrocarbons (PAHs).

The world of endocrine disruptors has been especially rife with regrettable substitutions. During the last few decades, one phthalate, DEHP, was replaced with another, DINP, while one type of flame retardant, PBDE, was replaced with another, Polymeric FR, and bisphenol A was replaced with bisphenol S. All of them turned out to be as—if not more—toxic to humans as what they replaced.

Take DINCH, which the chemical company BASF promoted as the "trusted non-phthalate plasticizer" for plastic in things like toys and food. When researchers compared the number of eggs retrieved from women during IVF to the amount of DINCH in the women's urine, they retrieved far fewer eggs from women with more DINCH.

And yes, whenever someone tests a fashion product, they seem to find at least one endocrine disruptor. In 2021, a lab found formaldehyde, aniline, and PFAS on surgical masks at the height of the pandemic, which means millions of people could have spent the pandemic breathing in PFAS. (Which might also, by the way, suppress the immune system.) In 2021, the Center for Environmental Health in California found high levels of BPA in polyester-spandex socks by the brands Hanes, Champion, Tommy Hilfiger, New Balance, Fruit of the Loom, Reebok, Forever 21, and many more, at up to nineteen times California's safe limit. In 2022, CEH tested sports bras, and found similarly high levels of BPA in those sold by Athleta, PINK, Asics, North Face, Brooks, All in Motion, Nike, and FILA. And when the Canadian Broadcasting Corporation had thirty-eight pieces of children's clothing tested from ultra-fast-fashion brands Zaful, AliExpress, and Shein, it found that one in five had elevated levels of toxic chemicals like lead, PFAS, and phthalates. A Shein toddler jacket and red purse contained almost twenty times and five times, respectively, the limit for lead in California and Canada. When H&M and IKEA had secondhand clothing from around the world tested in 2021, they found APEOs in almost all the wool samples and traces of chromium in almost 9 percent of the samples—and this is after these products had most likely been worn, washed, and donated.

Polyester is also at risk for containing antimony, which is added during production to speed up the production process. In 2022, the Maine-based nonprofit Defend Our Health found that 40 percent of the beverages in PET plastic bottles that it tested from major brands contained concentrations of antimony above 1 part per billion, California's public health goal for contaminants in drinking water. PET plastic bottles are the ones that are recycled into polyester for eco-friendly brands. And antimony is the heavy metal that Renaissance Italians used in their poison recipes, alongside arsenic, lead, and mercury. It has shown up multiple times in airline uniforms, in household dust, and in higher amounts in children's urine than in adults'.

Industry folks often roll their eyes at these tests. *Fearmongering*, they call them. During a 2021 webinar on toxic fashion chemistry for fashion-brand employees, a presenter talked about Greenpeace's 2013 Little Monsters campaign, which found nonylphenol ethoxylates (NPEs, a subset of APEOs), phthalates, organotins, PFAS, and antimony in children's clothing sold worldwide from brands including Disney, Gap, H&M, Uniqlo, Adidas, Nike, Puma, and Burberry. "Some of the chemicals that they found were within the legal limit, but they published it anyway," the presenter said.

By 2013, we understood there is no safe level of endocrine disruptors, especially when it comes to children. Regulators may have been slow to catch up, but it doesn't mean Greenpeace was incorrect to call these brands out.

This isn't just a concern for couples who want to start a family. Girls are maturing and getting their periods earlier, which is associated with increased risk of type 2 diabetes, asthma, and breast cancer. There's evidence that conditions like polycystic ovary syndrome (PCOS), endometriosis, and fibroids are becoming more common, and a 2021 study out of Spain showed women who reported high use of cosmetics like hair spray, face creams, hair dyes, and lipsticks had higher levels of endocrine-disrupting chemicals, and higher rates of endometriosis.

More children are being born with intersex, ambiguous, or malformed genitalia. Male infertility is associated with increased risk of heart disease, plus testicular and prostate cancer, and overall higher mortality rates. A study that Swan was involved in found that premenopausal women who had the most of the phthalate DEHP in their urine were more likely to lack interest in sex.

Unfortunately, many fertility doctors are also rolling their eyes. "I have talked to providers that are like, yeah, I just don't think it's really a big deal," the North Carolina–based fertility doctor Ashley Eskew told me. She cofounded OvulifeMD—a website that provides evidence-based dietary, environmental, and lifestyle modification suggestions to women who struggle to conceive or have experienced multiple miscarriages—with her husband, board-certified integrative medicine physician Will Haas.

"I mention it at every single first patient encounter that I have, and they are like, *I had no idea.* So I think that there is still a big gap, both in training in this area to help providers understand, hey, it does matter, and then also to disseminate that to their patients," Eskew told me.

"The good news is, especially in the case of BPA and that sort of thing, they have a short half-life. So small changes that you make today will result in a difference tomorrow or the next day or the next day." It's true. Bisphenols like BPA and phthalates are water soluble—we pee them out fairly quickly. If our exposure completely stopped today, they would be mostly gone within a week. But we are exposed to them from such a wide variety of places on such a regular basis, their levels in the average American body stay about the same. Heavy metals and PFAS, that "forever chemical," on the other hand, are persistent, building up in our fat and hanging out doing their damage for years and years. The quicker we can stop our exposure to them, the better. We'd better start now.

"The big ones that we talked about, like phthalates, BPA, lead, heavy metals, all of those things add up over time," Eskew said. "If we get a small amount from our food, and if we get a small amount from our clothes, and we get a small amount from our personal care products, then what does that look like at the end of the day? That additive effect, if you actually looked at that, then I guarantee that all of these things would be high enough to cause some sort of symptom and problem. But we've normalized that. How much of today's society has normalized feeling fatigued? Or having dry, itchy skin, or having some sort of reactive asthma to something, like, *Oh, well, I just wheeze sometimes*, like not actually investigating that further?"

It's anecdotal, but Eskew has noticed that a lot of her patients, more than in the general population, have autoimmune thyroiditis (Hashimoto's disease), where immune antibodies attack their own thyroid, causing all sorts of health problems, like fatigue, constipation, and hair loss. The upshot is that in the process of detoxifying so they can start a family, they see other health problems clear up, too. "You do tend to see a higher incidence of some of these sorts of things in certain patients—atopic dermatitis, asthma, other reactive airway diseases. Then you realize, more often than not, it's some environmental insult. You remove that insult, and it's like a new person, a new patient altogether. So I definitely think that there's a big link there," she said.

As I would find later, Eskew's not the only one seeing a link between chemicals and autoimmune disease.

Disrupting the Disruptors

When I later asked Candice if she had any other health issues, she said "only" what she thinks was eczema and some digestive issues from childhood.

A no-nonsense brunette with a slight Texas twang, Candice got into making fused glass art in a kiln in her studio after she met her husband, and worked with polyurethane and burned wood to make some decorative signs.

"I was just completely clueless, living the life any normal person who doesn't know would probably be living," she said. She bought drugstore personal care products for herself and her husband. She loved junk food, and they took advantage of living in the city to eat out at fast-food restaurants.

She wasn't a big fashion person; she still buys and gets most of her clothing from stores like Marshalls, Ross, and JCPenney or secondhand. Her husband, however, is a big fan of quick-dry outdoor gear, which—unless it explicitly says it doesn't—has a PFAS-based durable water repellent.

By the time they got married, they hadn't used protection for three years but had never gotten pregnant. So they consulted a doctor, and after running some tests, he said that together they had just a 4 percent chance of getting pregnant without medical intervention. The problem likely lay with both their bodies, they were told. After eight months of trying and praying, they decided they would have to take the help. She started a medication to induce ovulation, but still, nothing happened.

They had just moved across the state, deep cleaning their rental with the strongest cleaners available at the supermarket before they left so they could get their deposit back. They moved into a home with new carpeting and giant windows that they covered with new blackout curtains with pungent vinyl backing. They bought a new memory-foam bed.

When her husband got his graduate degree, they moved back home to a small town two hours away from the nearest clinic. The fertility doctor at that clinic told them it was time to try IVF.

"And it's honestly the three letters I never really wanted to hear, because I know that for one, it's extremely expensive, and taxing on your body," Candice said. "I was desperate to become a mother." They didn't have the money for it, so her in-laws lent them the $18,000. That made the news that the first whole round had failed even worse.

"You know, a lot of patients struggle so much with anxiety and depression when they're diagnosed with infertility," said Eskew. "Studies have shown it's been comparable to that of a cancer diagnosis for patients." When she speaks to patients about detoxifying, she says, "I try to phrase it in a way that it's like, this should be empowering because this is something that you *do* have control over."

In Candice's case, finding the book *It Starts with the Egg* did give her a feeling of control over what previously had felt like a complete gamble. (I actually found her by posting in a Facebook group for acolytes of *ISWTE*.) She threw out all her cleaning products, all their personal care products, and anything else that had "fragrance" in the ingredient list. She purged her kitchen of packaged and processed food, and plastic containers. She bought organic produce and grass-fed meat.

"Of course we didn't really have the money, but we also couldn't afford not to," she told me. "I changed anything that touched my body or his."

Well, except fashion. She hadn't heard that fashion can also have endocrine disruptors. In fact, neither had Eskew until I emailed her links to news stories and studies on the topic.

"I mean, whenever I got your email, I was like, 'Will [her husband], can you believe this?'" Eskew told me. "I just felt so uninformed and out of the loop. Why aren't we talking about this in the medical community either? We're looking at it in all of these other things, from the dust we bring into the house, to the flame retardant that's on your couch, to the creams and lotions. But what about what's touching your skin all day every day? Like, why hasn't this come up yet?

"The children's clothing, that's the thing that got me as well," she said, about the tests of children's clothing from Shein and Zaful. "One of the pictures that was in one of the articles that you linked to, it's a dress with a princess on it, which is the exact dress that I sent my niece for her birthday. And I mean, that's an especially high-risk population.

"It is deeply disturbing, I think, to not have an ingredient label on your clothes, once you realize all of these things are in there."

To pay for the second round, Candice's family managed to scrape together the $12,000 cost (a discount!) through a combination of selling cattle and staging a garage sale of old furniture. Despite the financial strain it put on the family, Candice felt good about this time.

"That one just felt right, it wasn't as stressful," she said. They managed to get nine eggs, which was disappointing. But that night she got a call from the doctor, who said four were mature and three had fertilized. She was thrilled. "That means that from the first round, I had a 20 percent fertilization rate. And the second round after changing my lifestyle for those four months before ovulation, I had a 75 percent fertilization rate." With only nine eggs, if her rate had been the same as the first round, she likely would have gotten nothing.

Six weeks later, on Valentine's Day, they heard their son's heartbeat for the first time. He was born in the fall of 2017, weighing just over eight pounds and perfectly healthy.

A couple of years later, they decided to try one more time, and she refined her diet and detox plan, switching to organic underwear as well.

This time, when she went in, they got twenty-one eggs, with

fourteen mature and a 100 percent fertilization rate. She had twins. And she credits it all to her work detoxifying her life.

"I think the most gratifying thing of Ovulife," Eskew said, "has been that women, no matter the outcome on their journey—and we never promised pregnancy—but they're like, *I'm living a better lifestyle than I ever have. And I feel better than I ever did.* And that is what it's all about, right?"

Candice doesn't just feel healthier. She has found her purpose. She started a Facebook community to share her story and is training to become a fertility coach with a focus on nontoxic living.

"I'm so thankful that my eyes have been opened to all the toxins, because now I can protect my baby from those," she said.

Oh, and the cherry on top? Her skin condition went away.

CHAPTER 6

YOU'RE JUST TOO SENSITIVE

The Mysterious Realm of Chemical Intolerance

Chingy Wong came back to her hotel from dinner at her go-to Thai restaurant in Dublin, where she had a layover. She decided to try on her new uniform to make sure it was wrinkle-free and fit well. She pulled the mock turtleneck over her head and slipped on the skirt, then buttoned the purple sweater on top.

As she played with tying the scarf around her neck, a wave of nausea rolled over her. She wondered if she had food poisoning or was coming down with a cold. But when she took off the uniform and lay down, she felt better within a half hour.

Chingy had heard about the uniform troubles at Alaska Airlines but hadn't thought much of it. "I thought it was just their allergies," she told me. She wasn't worried because she wasn't allergic to anything. Yet.

The next morning, she put the uniform back on, but this time over an undershirt and control-top pantyhose. Throughout her flight back to JFK, she felt slightly nauseated, dizzy, and hot. Her heart palpitated even as she stood in the galley, catching her breath.

It was May 29, 2018, and all over the world, from Huntsville to Honolulu, Spokane to Sydney, Delta employees were donning their new designer uniforms by Zac Posen. "It was an honor to design for an iconic global aviation brand and I wanted to bring back glamour to the runway while introducing innovative technologies in the uniforms," Posen said in a Delta press release.

Attendants were also asking for textile technology. "My biggest concern was that there would be a stain-resistant factor and that the uniforms would be fairly wrinkle-free," a longtime Delta flight attendant who was on the uniform feedback committee told the *New York Times*.

Best of all, the airline had no reason to fear the health issues happening at other airlines. These uniforms were made by Lands' End, the higher-end brand that both American and Alaska had entrusted to make safer replacement uniforms.

Many Delta attendants weren't a fan of the signature passport-plum dress—they called it Barney purple. An older attendant told me that she thought it was too sexy, like what Barbie would wear to serve Ken in first class—and not designed for attendants who had larger bodies. But Chingy, twenty-nine years old and slim, with long, shiny black hair, loved it. "I thought it was really cute," she said.

Anyway, she had known worse. Chingy had been born in Hong Kong and raised in Chicago, and one of her first jobs was at the Hong Kong–based airline Cathay Pacific, which required attendants to wear heels, stay under a certain weight, and take classes in makeup and hairstyling. An LPD (little purple dress) was something she could handle, as long as she could wear comfortable shoes.

There was an off note, however. When she pulled the new uniform pieces out of the box at her home (now in Ohio), the smell of chemicals, acrid and faintly sweet, hit her. The fabric was also cheaper and thinner than the uniform she had been fitted for a month earlier. Could it be this cheap, smelly uniform that was causing her health problems on her first flight in it?

When she finally got home from Dublin, after her flight to JFK and commuter flight to Ohio, she washed the uniform several times. That seemed to resolve the problem, mostly. She still got a runny nose when she worked, and she was always sneezing. But she was handling it okay. She was young! Not like the older attendants who had been working on airplanes for decades. Her body was resilient, or so it seemed.

By that November, Chingy had washed the uniform so many times that the dye had faded. So she asked Delta to send her a new uniform. "And that one stinked to high heaven," she said. "That was worse than my first one. It smelled so bad." Her chest turned red and burned, and her hands started shaking. Her memory started failing—she would have to ask passengers to repeat their drink orders. She wondered whether she was getting Parkinson's.

That's when she was invited to join a Facebook group that the flight attendant Heather Poole at American Airlines had started for all the attendants at the four different airlines who were going through similar ordeals. There, she saw pictures of rashes so bad the spots were purple and bleeding, and of bald spots on female attendants' heads. There were tales of severe sinus infections, nosebleeds, swollen eyes, fainting spells, and blood in urine. One mother reported that her baby developed a rash on his cheek after he had nursed while she was wearing the skirt. The menace wasn't completely invisible—the Barney-purple Delta uniforms had a tendency to bleed and stain attendants' skin (and sheets, and bras, and bathtubs) purple.

Chingy now had allergies. On a commuter flight, she was sitting next to a passenger wearing perfume, and had to run to the bathroom to vomit. She went to a dermatologist at Ohio State University, who did a skin patch test that showed she was allergic to formaldehyde and nickel. Then she went to a pulmonologist, who diagnosed her with adult-onset asthma. He put her in a chamber with the uniforms and found that her breathing became restricted. Both he and a dermatologist told her she shouldn't wear the uniforms anymore.

Delta granted her request to wear a black uniform and white

shirt she bought herself, but on her next flight in March to London, as she worked alongside other attendants in the crowded galley, her vertigo got so bad she could barely stand up. Her eyeballs burned; her upper stomach contracted in pain. She walked to the front of the plane, away from her coworkers, and felt better, but when an attendant approached her, she started coughing, as if something were stuck in her throat.

When they landed and she had to pile onto a bus with other attendants and pilots to go to the hotel, exhaustion overtook her. She told her coworker she didn't feel well. He looked at her, the color completely drained from her face, and agreed. They went to the ER together.

"I felt like that was like the end of my career. I saw it coming," Chingy said. Delta flew her back to the United States a day later as a passenger, and on a conference call told her they were grounding her. She hasn't flown since.

A Perplexing—and Controversial—Diagnosis

Chingy's life became severely restricted by her reactions to scents and chemicals. Visiting the grocery store made her sick, and she threw out her scented detergent.

She had developed what is diagnosed variously as multiple chemical sensitivity, environmental illness, mast cell activation syndrome, or toxicant-induced loss of tolerance. That what Chingy was going through doesn't yet have one widely accepted name reflects the fact that it's not a widely accepted diagnosis in the medical community. And there's no code a doctor can write for insurance.

Triggered by overexposure to toxins, those with chemical intolerance are exquisitely attuned to the introduction of toxins and chemicals into their environment. Like human Geiger counters, they react violently to the kinds of things that for the rest of us might cause only a headache, if it bothers us at all: a colleague's strong perfume, that "new car smell," or a freshly painted wall.

The foundation of this theory—that many illnesses and allergies are the result of everyday exposure to modern synthetic chemicals—was first put forth in the 1940s by a maverick allergist, Dr. Theron G. Randolph. With a degree from University of Michigan Medical School, a fellowship at Harvard Medical School, and professorship at Northwestern, he wasn't exactly a quack. But his unorthodox views were never quite accepted by the medical establishment, even though he founded several popular synthetic-chemical-free recovery facilities for patients and led a nationwide movement of doctors who provided treatment for environmental illness. At the time of Randolph's death in 1995, Dr. Martha White, director of research at the Institute for Asthma and Allergy at Washington Hospital Center, told the *New York Times*, "The issue of being allergic to the environment is viewed with skepticism and is unproven."

Even as White pooh-poohed this theory, Gulf War syndrome, a mysterious illness with a constellation of unexplained symptoms, was cropping up. Characterized by chronic fatigue, cognitive problems, fibromyalgia, skin rashes, digestive issues, muscle and joint pain, and respiratory disorders, this illness was present in one-third of the soldiers who fought in the 1991 Gulf War. Doctors cannot identify the exact cause: pesticide exposure, oil-well fires, chemical weapons, or burn pits—or some combination—could have been the culprit.

Media interest in what at the time was called multiple chemical sensitivity (MCS) crested in the late nineties before undergoing an almost systematic discrediting. Most women I talked to who exhibited symptoms of chemical intolerance, like Debbie in Gloversville, had never heard of MCS. Neither is it well known among communities of color, Rachel Lee, professor of English and gender studies at the Institute for Society and Genetics at UCLA, told me.

She led a project where she and her students interviewed women who suffer from MCS, but they had a hard time finding participants. One Latino student said his own mom had never heard of MCS, but she did have asthma attacks when confronted with strong smells.

"Generally, in a primary-care setting in a standard conventional family medicine practice, you don't see a lot of patients that are 'chemically sensitive,'" Dr. Elizabeth Seymour at the Environmental Health Center in Dallas told me. "They may say, *I don't like smells*, or something."

Seymour sees patients who have already spent thousands of dollars going from doctor to doctor, looking for the reason for their brain fog, headaches, fatigue, rashes, asthma, and fibromyalgia, a mysterious illness of musculoskeletal pain and fatigue.

"A lot of physicians and providers steer clear of these people because they're so complicated. There's seven pages worth of medical history and twenty or fifty diagnoses and symptoms," she says. "They usually will present with a history of *I was exposed to this*, or *I didn't know I was exposed to this, and I started getting a lot of symptoms*. And you have to be Sherlock Holmes and investigate."

Many allergists still don't understand how synthetic chemicals can cause these reactions. When Chingy went to an allergist and said she thought the uniform was the cause, the nurse practitioner laughed at the idea. Not long after, Chingy ended up in the ER with an anaphylactic attack—hives, closed throat—after she pulled the turtleneck over her head and face.

Because doctors can't see proof of chemical intolerance and its symptoms, it's often characterized as a physical manifestation of anxiety or depression, and patients get referred to a psychologist for treatment. (The fact that women are most often afflicted by chemical intolerance surely doesn't help doctors believe their ailments, either.)

"This is a problem in occupational health. We're dealing with people with psychological symptoms," Dr. Claudia S. Miller, an allergist, immunologist, and professor emerita at the University of Texas, told me. "They have a reaction where they get confused, they can't think. And so there's a tendency to say, well, that person's just depressed or anxious, when in fact, exposures are responsible for their symptoms. If your physicians don't believe you, that's the worst. Because then your coworkers, your employer, your family start to not believe you, either."

The main reason doctors hesitate to give a diagnosis of chemical intolerance is that there isn't a good biomarker they can point to. For regular allergies like pet dander or peanuts, we create antibodies in response to exposure, and those antibodies can be picked up in a blood test.

"Allergists like me, in my training, learn how to interview people and then test them for those kinds of allergies with a blood test or with a skin test," Miller said. "It's relatively straightforward."

But there's another part of the immune system whose inner workings, until recently, were somewhat of a mystery. Called cell-mediated immunity, it involves mast cells, an ancient protective mechanism that has been in our bodies since before we were human, a half a billion years ago. "It's the earliest and most basic immune response that we have," Miller said.

Researchers have begun to understand only in the past decade how mast cells function. Like archers positioned in the windows of a fortress, they are everywhere your tissue is in contact with the external environment: your skin; your digestive system, which processes food; your blood-brain barrier; and your lungs, which suck in outside air. When mast cells encounter something foreign that they don't like, whether bacteria or poison, they release packets of natural body chemicals called *cytokines*, which recruit the immune system to that place of incursion. This response causes inflammation wherever they feel the body is under attack, which can manifest as a rash, gut pain, asthma, brain fog, or other symptoms.

The thing is, mast cells can be sensitized. If they've been

overwhelmed once by a substance, they're on high alert—sort of like a traumatized soldier who, having been under fire, has a panic attack when he hears a bang. Likewise, when mast cells encounter just a hint of the same or a similar substance, they can freak out (*activate*) and release the cytokines again en masse, leading to an inflammatory response way out of proportion to the inciting substance. This looks like someone giving you a hug, sniffing, and then backing away with apologies and coughing because you use a scented laundry product. They may say they have to go lie down, or even leave.

"Once [mast cells] become sensitized, it takes a minute—I mean, *tiny*—exposure to trigger them to react. And they can react in a way that affects the entire body," Miller said.

One well-known example of cell-mediated immunity is poison ivy. I was exposed to poison ivy and its oil, urushiol, when I was a little child tromping around in the woods around our house in North Carolina. My first exposure wasn't bad; I just got a little rash. But every time after that, when I came into contact with poison ivy, I would be down for days afterward. Once, when I was nine years old, my face swelled up so large that my eyes squeezed shut. I managed to avoid poison ivy for twenty-two years, until I was on a small lake island in Nicaragua covered in mango trees that dropped their fruit all over the ground. I ended up with rashes all over my ankles. Turns out, mango skin also has urushiol.

"That's cell-mediated immunity; that's *memory* of that poison ivy," Miller explained.

This two-step process is why she has given it the diagnostic name *toxicant-induced loss of tolerance*, or TILT. First, the initial exposure event—whether new carpeting, mold, harsh cleaning products, pesticides, the smoke from a wildfire that's burning up plastic-filled homes, or a toxic uniform—sensitizes someone to a substance. From then on, just a tiny bit of exposure will set them off. And Miller's research shows that chemical intolerance is a function of mast cell activation.

Furthermore, Miller believes that mast cell activation can happen in response to not just the initial trigger but all sorts of synthetic chemicals and scents. "We really don't have all the answers yet. But it's clear that once the mast cells are activated, then they can be triggered by structurally- and chemically-unrelated substances," she said. So if you were triggered by mold and its toxic volatile organic compounds, you might then be sensitive to *all* scented products and volatile organic compounds.

Miller calls out fossil fuel products specifically as something our bodies have not evolved to deal with. The production of chemicals created from fossil fuels, such as pesticides and polymers, exploded after World War II, which is also when Dr. Theron G. Randolph started his practice of treating environmental illness. (Perhaps it should have been called "synthetic illness.") But dyes made from coal tar, I told Miller, became ubiquitous long before that, in the late 1800s, causing all sorts of skin problems. Still, an extra fifty years is not enough for our bodies to adapt to such high and daily exposure.

Chingy got tested and found out she's super allergic to formaldehyde "on a microscopic level," plus benzene (the toxic chemical used to make dyes), nickel, and acetone. Just a tiny amount of these substances made her immune system—and those of Heather Poole from American Airlines and other flight attendants I spoke to—go into overdrive, temporarily disabling them and making it impossible for them to work.

The problem is, as Miller pointed out, the amount of a chemical that disables people who are chemically intolerant is far below what toxicologists have defined as the safe level of exposure for most chemicals. Toxicologists come up with that safe level by exposing rats or mice or other animals to a decreasing amount of the chemical until there is "no observed adverse effect" on the animal. Then they divide that amount by a factor of ten to a thousand to be safe, and transpose that to the average human's body weight. Note, though, it's an *observable* effect. "Animals usually can't tell you if they're having trouble with concentration and memory, that they have brain fog," Miller says. "They can't tell you if they are having problems tolerating their foods.

"The problem that patients face is that once TILT is developed, the things that trigger their symptoms, the levels are far lower than the levels that the toxicologists come up with. And so, when they go to court over something like, let's say, the chemicals that are in the clothing, then the toxicologists have their interpretation . . . They will look at the person's exposure, whether it's industrial exposure or some other exposure, and say, well, the levels of exposure are far below the 'no observable adverse effect level' that we've tested in animal studies."

And so, the attendants are effectively told that what is happening to them is not possible.

All in Your Head . . . and Your Skin, and Your Throat

Chemical intolerance has been linked to many types of chemical overexposure: new homes and new workplace buildings with fresh paint and carpets, indoor pesticide exposure, and mold. Many patients believe it was long- term low- level exposures, or overlapping exposures from different things, like mold followed by fresh flooring and walls.

While toxic fashion isn't commonly identified as a precursor, the chemical intolerant do find themselves reacting to toxic clothing. A 1995 study of thirty-five people who had developed chemical sensitivity through their work showed that 86 percent of them had changed the type of clothing they wore, to cope.

Seymour at the Environmental Health Center has a variety of tests at her disposal that use urine, blood, and hair samples to look for toxic chemicals like solvents and heavy metals that might be causing the symptoms. But if a patient presents with a rash only in a certain area, she often starts asking about the clothing they are wearing or the detergent they are using.

Unfortunately, pinpointing an allergy is less than half the battle. When it comes to clothing, which doesn't have an ingredient list, how can you avoid formaldehyde or disperse blue? "It's becoming more difficult to avoid these chemicals," Seymour said. "There are multiple chemicals that are put in everything. And your clothing is included in that."

I talked to several women who suffer from chemical intolerance, asking them about what they had to do to avoid reacting to clothing, hoping that it would reveal something about what invisible menace is on there. "No chemically sensitive person does dry cleaning," said Dr. Ann McCampbell, who worked in a gynecology clinic at UC Santa Barbara before she became ill in 1989. (She's not sure what caused it.) Now she does phone consultations for people who react to chemicals.

"Some people are naked in their houses because they can't tolerate clothes anymore," she said. "The really sick ones are all swaddled in white or beige, because the dyes are too much usually." She said one client has eczema and can't do even 2 percent spandex in her clothing, and she described people hanging new clothing outside for months in the sun and rain, stuffing it in a pressure cooker, and soaking it in powdered milk and vinegar. Some people will buy athletic sneakers and put them outside for three years, hoping they'll eventually be able to wear them.

For a while, McCampbell would go to yard sales for used clothing, plus Goodwill and thrift stores until some started using scents like Febreze on everything. "I couldn't really tolerate new clothes for quite a while. Now I can get a white T-shirt from Walmart and wash it a few times and it'll be okay," she said. A few years back, she wanted black jeans to play in her rock 'n' roll band, so she went to a discount store and bought some. "It was horrible, they just stunk. I got a headache. It almost ruined the washing machine."

She's actually able to tolerate a wrinkle-resistant shirt she bought. But stain-repellent and water-resistant outdoor gear? Forget about it. "Tents are impossible," she said. She recently bought Patagonia shorts and the elastic in the band did her in. A T-shirt with a vinyl print on the front she couldn't tolerate, either.

TILT researcher Claudia Miller has been in conversation with Judith Anderson of the Association of Flight Attendants, and the attendants' experience makes sense to her. "Often, if they're in tight quarters, and they're around other people that have uniforms, it would make sense to me that you have those tiny fibers that get airborne, or even the volatile chemicals in the garments, and then the person has a common reaction like an asthma attack," she said.

Even though the sensitization can be experienced in a half dozen different body systems, the skin is the only place doctors can easily identify it, through patch tests, like the ones that the airline attendants and Jaclyn, the New York fashion production manager with Crohn's, got.

Most of these patch tests involve only around eighty substances, because that is all that can fit on someone's back. But there are many, many more substances a dermatologist could order from a company that makes patch tests, and thousands more substances beyond that which could be in a garment. Many of these fashion chemicals, as we saw at Duke, have never actually been cataloged, much less distilled into a sample. "Some people have found it easier just to take the material itself that they suspect the person may be reacting to, and make that into a patch test," Miller said.

If that fabric does cause a reaction, for the purposes of holding a uniform maker accountable, you have to figure out which exact chemical in that fabric caused the reaction, then demonstrate that, by itself, the chemical causes the exact debilitating symptoms someone has. That is a virtually impossible task.

Even though it's not as talked about today as it was in the 1990s, the number of people diagnosed with chemical sensitivity increased 300 percent from 2006 to 2016. But it might be far more prevalent than diagnoses would have you believe. Miller's research team has administered a fifty-question test called the QEESI that represents that international reference standard, and their shorter version called BREESI, to ten thousand Americans. It asks respondents to rate how sick things like perfumes, gasoline fumes, and paint thinners—as well as foods and medications—make them feel. More than 20 percent of respondents answered in a way that indicated they have a chemical intolerance. That number, 20 percent, lines up pretty well with the portion of attendants having reactions to their uniforms at the three airlines for which we have that data. It also lines up with the percentage of Americans who have suffered from contact dermatitis.

As I researched this book, I, too, began to grasp chemical intolerance's true prevalence. More often than not, when I told friends and acquaintances the topic of the book, they would share with me that they or a dear friend or family member can't tolerate scents. One woman whom I was about to hire to fact-check the book backed out because this topic hit too close to home—she herself is so intolerant of scented products and synthetic clothing that it has severely disrupted her life.

Miller has been working on this science for decades, but when I spoke to her in the fall of 2021, she still hadn't been able to push it out into the mainstream. "A lot of doctors don't even believe it," she said. "It's very hard for science to understand new information. There's a saying, something like, *The mind responds to new ideas the way the immune system responds to foreign materials.* Rejection is the first thing that happens in any kind of development of science."

"Normal" people who can breathe in gasoline fumes or fragranced detergents and go about their day see themselves as the rational ones. It's easier to believe all the experts who say not to worry, that it's handled, that anyone who reacts is just too sensitive, than to believe what these bodies of women are telling us.

But that might be changing. In November of 2021, Miller and her team published a paper in *Environmental Sciences Europe* titled "Mast cell activation may explain many cases of chemical intolerance." Because the peer-reviewed paper—which was sent out to toxicologists worldwide—links mast cell activation to TILT, it finally explains what is going on in our bodies, opening the door for doctors to understand and believe people who come to them asking for a diagnosis and help.

"If you don't have a biological mechanism, they don't believe it," Miller said to me a year after our first call. "And there was no biological mechanism to explain it until they learned about mast cells."

Now Miller is being invited to present at events on topics ranging from pesticides to the microbiome and autism. Whether and when this research will trickle down to the doctors tasked with treating the chemically intolerant—and the toxicologists asked to assess the health threat of chemical exposure—is a whole other question.

CHAPTER 7

ATTACKING OUR OWN BODIES

The Looming Autoimmune Epidemic

Tonya Osborne wrapped her hands around the cup of hot water, seeking relief for her sore joints. At sixty years old, she wondered whether she was finally succumbing to aging and getting arthritis. She hoped not; at the time, she had plans to keep flying until she reached her nineties.

But Southwest Airlines attendants don't push carts—they carry trays—and it was becoming quite painful for her to do the drinks service. Her back had started to hurt, too. And she thought Southwest also needed to clean the air vents on these planes. She had developed migraines and a sinus infection that would not go away. "My nose was running like a faucet," she told me later.

When she joined Southwest in 1999, Tonya was a forty-year-old divorced mother, and grateful for the opportunity to join a company famous for its culture that valued employees, all the way down to the attendants. She read the founder Herb Kelleher's book and took his axioms to heart, like "I'd rather have a company bound by love than a company bound by fear."

"We were like a family," she told me about her early days, when the attendants wore cargo shorts, white sneakers, and varsity sweaters with SWA in big letters down the front, all by the uniform maker Cintas. By the 2010s, though, the airline had expanded and been enormously profitable for decades, and Kelleher had long since retired—Gary Kelly took over as CEO in 2004.

The summer of 2017, Southwest Airlines debuted its kicky new uniforms. Stripes down the side of the dresses mimicked the bright new stripes painted on the body and tails of its airplanes. For these uniforms, the airline had switched from Lands' End back to Cintas.

Tonya didn't like the new uniforms, which were polyester. "Which is plastic," she told me over the phone in her charming Georgia drawl. "It's not good on an airplane. It does not breathe. And when you're on there and you're running up and down the aisle, say you've got a hot airplane, the AC is not working all that great, that uniform sticks to you."

In May of 2018, as she was getting off a plane, Tonya noticed red blotches on her skin around her chest and neck. They looked almost like sunburn spots. She went to her primary care doctor in Florida, where she now lived, who told her she had hives and wrote her a sick note and prescription for steroid cream. When they hadn't cleared up two days later, she sent Tonya to a dermatologist for a patch test. The resulting report said she was allergic to dyes. And her skin reaction was getting worse. "I'm telling you, they were like burns with blisters," she said. She submitted a doctor's note to Southwest, according to a report by the *Philadelphia Inquirer*, which said if she "continues to wear the uniform, she will continue to have a severe rash that may reduce her ability to perform her duties."

But she wasn't allowed to switch to a look-alike uniform. So she started paying other attendants to pick up her flights so she could have a break—$75 here, $150 there. It was adding up to thousands of dollars, but she had no choice. If she accrued too many absentee points, she would be fired.

In the end, it only delayed the inevitable. By the end of the summer, it became impossible for her to work. Her last day on a plane was August 31, and she went on what she hoped was temporary leave. Not long after, her landlord sold her rental home out from under her, and she couldn't qualify for a home loan to buy a place. So she moved into a friend's RV. But she figured this was temporary. Once the uniforms were gone, she could go back to work and get back on her feet.

A month later, Sonya Lacore, Southwest's vice president of In-flight Operations, sent out an email to the attendants. "I'm pleased to share that Southwest recently had all of the flight attendant uniform pieces tested to reinforce our confidence in the fabrics and materials. Our uniform supplier and Southwest each had the test results evaluated by independent medical experts who confirmed that employees are not subject to health hazards when wearing the uniform garments and accessories."

Tonya shot off an email to Lacore, plus any other executive at Southwest with a fancy title, requesting to see the toxicology report.

"This situation has caused a great deal of physical, financial and emotional stress," she wrote. "Immediate action needs to be taken so that we do not have to wait until next year to get the proper tools we need to come to work without being sick. I know Southwest wants this company represented at the very best. I feel you are trying. I don't think anyone realizes how many of us are battling reactions in different forms, and some not realizing what's causing their illnesses. I don't understand why, when there's flight attendants out here that want and need to work that someone can't figure something out to give us the proper tools to work with that will not be harmful to us."

Southwest called her to Dallas for a meeting at headquarters, where she was handed a sheet with a pass-fail chart that listed "dyes and other dyestuffs" and "allergens." But when she asked what the "other dyestuffs" were and for more information about the substances marked as "fail," she couldn't get a straight answer. While she took notes, an employee leaned over her to watch. She wasn't allowed to keep a copy of the vague report.

"The test results are entirely consistent with what would be expected if similar off-the-rack retail garments were tested," a spokesperson for the uniform maker, Cintas, said.

Tonya told a reporter at the *Philadelphia Inquirer* that, as she remembers it, during the meeting, a company executive said Southwest and Cintas didn't want to scuttle the $11 million uniform contract. They preferred to run through all the current stock of uniforms before switching them out. (I reached out to Southwest Airlines for comment, but they did not respond.)

Unfortunately, though Tonya and Judith Anderson at the AFA spoke over email, Anderson could do very little to help her. Southwest's attendants are represented by Transport Workers Union Local 556, a small union in Texas just for SWA attendants that was incorporated in 1981. Back then, ironically, it was also a uniform issue that drove attendants to organize—their year-round uniform involved hot pants, which invited sexual harassment from male passengers. (They ended up winning the ability to wear a wrap skirt over the pants.)

But in 2020, the union seemed outmatched by the airline. When a reporter from the *Philadelphia Inquirer* asked, the union declined to share the exact number of attendants who reported reactions, only saying "hundreds" of its members reported skin reactions, swelling, headaches, and breathing problems. It was trying to get a reporting system up and running.

One Southwest flight attendant who started losing her hair managed to get answers by sending her uniform to a private lab for testing. The results showed benzyl alcohol, which is used as a dye carrier and can cause skin and breathing problems, plus elevated levels of fourteen heavy metals, including chromium, arsenic, mercury, and lead. "The levels in these compounds will cause severe allergic reactions to the individual wearing the clothing," the toxicologist said, including "asthma, bronchitis, or even chemically induced pneumonia."

The year 2019 did not bring Tonya relief. She emptied out her

401(k) and the rest of her profit-sharing proceeds from Southwest to buy her own RV, pay for medical expenses, and pay for living expenses. She had surgeries on her hand, arm, and rotator cuff. "It's amazing how much your body all of a sudden just starts falling apart," she quipped to me.

When the article about Tonya's lopsided battle against Southwest came out in the *Philadelphia Inquirer*, on March 7, 2020, it caused barely a ripple. That same day, the governor of New York issued a state of emergency order because of COVID-19. But Dr. Graham Peaslee from the University of Notre Dame offered to test six of Tonya's pieces for free. He found chromium, nickel, zinc, and bromine, which indicated to him that there might be brominated flame retardants. (Or perhaps, we now know given Duke's research on house dust, brominated azobenzene disperse dyes?)

"Also, when I was unpacking the garments, there were definitely organic odors associated with some of the garments, so I think there's some volatile organic compounds. We don't really test for those here," Peaslee wrote. His tests wouldn't hold up in a court of law, he told Tonya, especially since his lab wasn't certified. The results were just meant to show her which items she should get tested at a pricier, certified lab—and reassure her that she wasn't crazy, that there was something there. Even if she was never able to point to the one thing. And even if Southwest refused to acknowledge it.

Not long after, Tonya was diagnosed with psoriatic arthritis, a type of arthritis linked with psoriasis, a chronic skin disease. She also developed ankylosing spondylitis, which can eventually cause some of the bones in the vertebrae to fuse together. When I spoke to her in the fall of 2021, she was taking eight pills of a medicine called methotrexate every Friday. "And every other Tuesday I give myself a shot of Humira, to manage the pain and to slow down the process," she said.

These are autoimmune diseases, which means technically their causes are unknown. But Tonya knew why this was happening: it was the uniforms. "My rheumatologist I think has in his records that based on everything that we've run across, it is highly likely that the uniforms caused these autoimmune illnesses," she told me. (She wasn't able to find me a copy of these records; he has sinced moved offices.)

That's why I've come back, yet again, to the airline uniforms. If there are regular women out there who can confidently connect their autoimmune disease to clothing covered with invisible, unlabeled chemicals, I have yet to find them.

Mutiny in the Body

For the past fifty years, the biomarkers for autoimmune disorders have been steadily rising. Some organizations have put the number of Americans with an autoimmune disease at twenty-four million, others at fifty million, which would make it more common than cancer or heart disease.

These estimates are imprecise because, while some of the eighty-plus autoimmune diseases such as type 1 diabetes, multiple sclerosis, lupus, and rheumatoid arthritis are well known, many are poorly defined and difficult to diagnose, sharing symptoms with many other conditions. There is no national autoimmune institute like there is for cancer and other diseases, and there is little funding for research to help us even begin to outline the problem. Often a diagnosis only collates a constellation of symptoms under one name, without ever providing any clarity on what caused the symptoms and how to ameliorate them.

The most conservative estimate I found puts autoimmune disease as the third-leading cause of chronic illness in America, affecting between 5 and 8 percent of the population. Most of these diseases have no cure and require lifelong treatment to ease symptoms.

Instances of children with inflammatory bowel disease and type

1 diabetes have recently shot up. But you could rightfully say this is a women's issue. About four-fifths of autoimmune patients are women, and autoimmune disease is the biggest cause of illness in women, according to AARDA, the Autoimmune Association. According to the 2008 book *The Autoimmune Epidemic*, by Donna Jackson Nakazawa, it shortens the average patient's life span by fifteen years.

All autoimmune diseases share one trait: the immune system, catalyzed by something, attacks a person's own body. For more than a decade, scientists have agreed that the *something* is in our environment: viruses and toxins.

Meghan O'Rourke, in her 2022 memoir *The Invisible Kingdom: Reimagining Chronic Illness*, wrote: "It is clear there is a genetic component to autoimmune diseases; they tend to cluster in families, and many people end up with more than one such disease. But it is also clear that environment plays a major role: cases of autoimmune disease are rising at almost epidemic rates in affluent Western countries." According to O'Rourke's reporting, twin studies suggest that autoimmune diseases are one-third genetic and two-thirds environmental.

The dominant theory is that while some people are genetically predisposed to autoimmune disease, their body needs to be hit with a high exposure to one or two things to develop it. In fact, research supports the theory that it's a one-two punch of a genetic predisposition and a virus or toxin that starts the downward spiral. "Examples of exposures associated with autoimmune diseases include infectious agents, pesticides, solvents, endocrine-disrupting chemicals, occupational exposure to respirable particulates and fibers, and personal factors such as cigarette-smoking history and diet preferences," a committee of top researchers and doctors wrote in their 2022 book *Enhancing NIH Research on Autoimmune Disease*.

"Now we're getting autoimmune diseases from Covid," Dr. DeLisa Fairweather, a contributor to the book and an associate professor of medicine and director of translational research for the Department of Cardiovascular Diseases at Mayo Clinic, told me. "That was from a viral infection, but we're doing it in a background of high chemical exposures in the US."

Even though researchers and doctors tend to study autoimmune diseases in a silo, the progression from allergy to full-blown illness, such as in Tonya's case, shows how interconnected all the systems of our bodies are.

Let's start with something basic: the breath. In 2017, 545 million people worldwide had a chronic respiratory disease, an almost 40 percent increase from 1990. Between 1980 and 2014, the US death rate from chronic respiratory diseases, such as COPD, interstitial lung disease, and pulmonary sarcoidosis, increased by nearly 30 percent—in 2015, before the pandemic, chronic respiratory diseases were the fifth-leading cause of death. COPD, which we encountered in Gloversville, is caused by inhaling irritants. At least 85 percent of COPD cases are currently related to smoking, but as smoking rates fall, researchers are linking COPD symptoms to allergens in household dust.

And there's a connection to infertility as well. Some doctors, according to Nakazawa's *The Autoimmune Epidemic*, estimate that up to a quarter of all women who suffer from recurrent pregnancy loss have antiphospholipid antibody syndrome (APS), alternately known as "sticky blood" or Hughes syndrome.

In general, people with autoimmune diseases, chemical sensitivity, chronic pain, chronic Lyme, Crohn's disease (like Jaclyn in New York), and long Covid are all caught in the middle of a debate about whether what they are experiencing is "real" and has a cause—or is in their head. I even listened to a dermatologist in Tirupur, the cotton-dyeing capital of India, tell me that his patients' eczema, including that of garment workers, was related only to stress and bad hygiene.

"Of the nearly 100 women I interviewed, all of whom were eventually diagnosed with an autoimmune disease or another concrete illness, more than 90 percent had been encouraged to seek treatment for anxiety or depression by doctors who told them nothing physical was wrong with them," O'Rourke wrote in her reported memoir. Other research showed that half of women are told nothing is wrong with them for *an average* of five years before receiving a diagnosis of an autoimmune disease.

Yes, there is some evidence that some forms of therapy can help patients work through the psychological impact of having such a disruptive illness, but research indicates that the disease markers stay the same. And anyway, before you can give a soldier therapy for his PTSD, you have to get him off the battlefield. In order to calm the body and remind it that it's not in danger, you first have to get it out of real danger.

The invisible interactions between the body and the mind are far more complex than saying it's all in the head. Something caused the immune system, the digestive system, the pain signals, the mast cells to go haywire. Multiple studies have established links between various autoimmune diseases and certain chemicals—that is not up for debate. A cluster of multiple sclerosis cases in El Paso, Texas, in the mid-nineties was linked to heavy metal pollution, for example, and there's evidence that endocrine disruptors like phthalates and BPA could be the reason why autoimmune diseases affect so many more women than men: because they influence our sex hormones. But even if it was a "real" physical thing that set these conditions off, by the time a doctor can be induced to look for it, the culprit has fled the scene, like a hit-and-run driver, leaving only unmeasurable brain fog and fatigue.

Fairweather revealed to me how this all works. As she explains it, we all have two types of immune responses: innate and adaptive. The *innate* response recognizes and fights infectious agents and toxins. The *adaptive* response builds a memory of what those infections and toxins look like and attacks them if they show up again. For example, for arthritis, having an innate response over and over to some invading toxin or virus can lead to an adaptive immune response that causes the painful and steady inflammation.

Involved in all these responses is the mast cell, that ancient guardian cell Dr. Claudia S. Miller told me is the biological explanation for TILT. "Historically, before we introduced all these chemicals into the world, [the mast cell's] main role was as an innate cell—one that recognizes all of the infectious organisms, like viruses and bacteria and parasites," Fairweather said. "Very importantly, it's the only one that recognizes toxins."

But the mast cell doesn't only recognize toxins or cause allergies. It's also involved in our adaptive response to help our immune system learn. "It's called immunological spread," she said. "That's how we gain better and better protection each time we're exposed to a virus like the flu. The immune response improves each time it sees the virus by recognizing more and more components of the virus."

That's how vaccines work: they're trained on a wee bit of harmless virus similar to the ones we want to be protected from, so that our body attacks things like smallpox or yellow fever.

But this immune system learning can work against us, especially in our toxin-filled world. Her example is a strawberry that always has the residue of a certain pesticide sprayed to kill strawberry-loving bugs. "The mast cell is going to target the chemical; the chemical is what is toxic. But because it keeps seeing the strawberry with the chemical over and over every time you eat it, it is eventually going to start responding to the strawberry. You're going to end up with a food allergy." This allergy can linger for anywhere from a few years to an entire lifetime—the only way to get rid of it is to avoid that toxin until your body's memory of its connection to strawberries fades.

I asked her if that might be why some women always react to polyester and other synthetics—because their body now associates polyester with certain toxins, like disperse dyes. She thought it sounded likely. "Maybe it's BPA, maybe it's this other dye, but they've made memory cells against whatever that is. And until those memory cells die, they're going to have a reaction. And the only way they can stop it is to completely not have any exposure to that. Only then would they be able to reintroduce that without having a reaction."

Without ingredient lists on fashion, how would someone with textile allergies pull that off?

It's not just the typical allergies, though. "The mast cell is unique in that it interacts with all of our major systems. It has a local response, it has a systemic response, it's affecting the nervous system, the hormone system, and the immune system," she told me. That explains how someone can get hives, brain fog, and fatigue all at the same time.

Fairweather is rare, because she has combined her research and clinical practice into chronic heart disease with the emerging research on autoimmune disease. "Part of the problem is that people who study these are siloed themselves. A lot of the patients will go to a specialist for their autoimmune disease. And those specialists are not used to having anything to do with mast cells or studying them. The other problem is that people that study inflammation and immune cells don't study mast cells. I'm unusual in that I'm mixing all the worlds together."

Talking to Fairweather, I finally understood why all the horror stories I heard about how clothes ruining someone's life always started with a rash or hives. They were warning signs. Distress signals. Cries for help. "I tell everybody that I have worked with regarding food allergies, that if you don't get this under control, this is going to manifest as some kind of chronic illness in your life," she said.

Unfortunately, a lot of this is cutting-edge research that is just now starting to connect the threads. "We don't have any good research or understanding of the role of chemicals in driving autoimmune diseases," Fairweather said. "Until we start getting research like that, and we show that the chemicals are causing problems, we're not going to have the sort of clout to go to the FDA or whoever and say, *We need to have these chemicals banned* or *We need to have these chemicals even monitored.* We have to show evidence that it is causing harm, before anything will be done."

In the spring of 2022, a committee Fairweather was a part of, the Committee for the Assessment of NIH Research on Autoimmune Diseases, recommended to Congress that a new office be created to coordinate and oversee funding for autoimmune research. It can't come soon enough. Our country's attitude toward chemicals so far has been *What doesn't kill you doesn't matter.* Unless a chemical can be connected definitively to cancer and death, we allow the poisonings to continue.

I don't know about you, but I don't just want to survive. I want to thrive. I want to live a long life free of mysterious pain. I want to have skin that is clear and not itchy. I want to have a well-functioning digestive system. I want to breathe clean and clear air, outdoors and in. I want to be free of weight fluctuations. I want to be full of energy. If I decide to have a baby, I want to do so without painful and expensive interventions. And then I want to be able to keep that baby safe and healthy, too.

"I miss it more than I ever could imagine," Tonya told me about working in the sky. "But I can't be around it." *It* meaning the chemicals on the uniforms.

Our grandparents and parents were told that we could achieve better living through chemistry. But maybe the best kind of life is achieved when we can say no to chemistry, especially chemistry that is created and applied to our clothing without our consent or knowledge.

PART IV

WHERE IT COMES FROM

CHAPTER 8

THE BELLY OF THE BEAST

The Reality of Textile Factories Abroad

"If you want to heal, you must quit your job," the doctor said.

Leelavathi was at the local health clinic, seeking help yet again for her skin problem. She was helplessly itchy, and cauliflower blisters had erupted on her arms and legs. She had consulted doctors from Tirupur, Erode, and Coimbatore, and tried traditional and Western medicines. Nothing helped. She wasn't sure how much longer she could keep going like this.

I met Leelavathi six months after this conversation with her doctor, in her neighbor's living room in Tirupur, in the state of Tamil Nadu, India. I was almost a year into my reporting. By that point, I'd interviewed dozens of scientists, researchers, and individuals dealing with chemicals in our clothing, and had experienced several times what I can only describe as exhilarating dismay as I made connections between chemicals, companies, and illness. If this were a murder mystery—and in a sense it was—my corkboard by now was covered with photos and names. It was thick with red yarn between them. I had the *who*, *what*, and *why*. What I didn't have was the *where* and *how*.

I knew from the beginning that almost all these textiles are now produced abroad, in places like India, Bangladesh, Turkey,

China, and Ethiopia. And I knew I needed to see the process of dyeing and finishing textiles for myself so I could truly understand—and show you—what is happening behind the curtain. More importantly, I wanted to meet the people working in the dyehouses and factories that make everything in our wardrobes, to hear directly from them whether they were experiencing the same sorts of effects from the chemicals that Western consumers experience. I had spoken over video with people across the United States. But the pandemic was easing and borders were opening again. It was time to get on a plane—three planes and a long car ride, to be exact.

Go look at your cotton T-shirts. Are some of them made in India? They were probably made in Tirupur (alternatively spelled Tiruppur). Specializing in cotton knitwear, such as T-shirts, for the Western market, it reportedly has around twenty-two thousand garment factories employing more than six hundred thousand workers. Its nickname is Dollar City, because so much foreign capital flows into its coffers. In 2022, the Tirupur Exporters' Association estimated the city would export $4.3 billion in knitwear, accounting for some 2.6 percent of the entire world's market share.

I could have visited any number of other more infamous (at least to Westerners) production hubs to investigate the chemicals used in fashion production: Bangladesh, Turkey, Vietnam, Pakistan, Indonesia, Morocco, or if I had been in the mood for some oppressive surveillance, China. (While I was in India, I met two journalists who had recently bowed to the inevitable and left China.) But researchers and local journalists and activists have produced reams of information in English publications on Tirupur's chemical saga.

I had been told by Dr. Siva Pariti, the senior technical marketing officer at BluWin, a global textile chemical auditing and consulting service, that the region that includes Tirupur is considered a regulatory success story. "You can't go to the south and say, *I want to see some colored canals.* It's not possible now," he said on a video call from his European office. "In the south of India, it is a mandatory requirement that 100 percent water be reused, and not a single drop of water should go out of your factory to the river. If it happens, you are closed. What happened, how transformation happened, how the courts intervened, how the small canals became rivers now, you can see it now in South India," Pariti told me. "Because seven years before, things were different." He said if I wanted to see dye units polluting with complete impunity, I should head to Panipat, north of Delhi, or join him for a visit to Bangladesh.

What he says is technically true. Tamil Nadu is a relatively progressive state—I saw several hammer-and-sickle symbols painted on walls while in Tirupur, denoting its communist history. The caste system's grip on society is looser here, and there is more social mobility, with many a garment worker's child growing up to be a doctor. An estimated 30 percent of all Tirupur textile workers are migrants from northern India who come here for economic opportunity.

But this economic opportunity has a dark side. In the late nineties, after three decades of growth in the city's manufacturing industry, the pollution became unbearable. The Noyyal River, which flows east through Coimbatore and the center of Tirupur, past the factories, was a dumping ground for sewage as well as untreated effluent from eight hundred dyehouses. That flowed down into a reservoir that had been built to serve farmers in 1992, turning it into a toxic lagoon of dead fish. A local activist showed me an impressive 2005 report put together as a school project by a group of Tirupur schoolgirls guided by their teacher, and it said that an estimated seventy-seven acres of farmland became unusable, the crops dying, the coconut palms drying up. The spiral-bound report had pictures of the girls in their school uniforms, standing with a farmer and peering down into the greasy black waters of one of what they estimated were almost five thousand agricultural wells contaminated with lead and cadmium. It also had photos of children who made the mistake of swimming in the water, their skin covered in blistered lesions and severe eczema. With the groundwater contaminated, two locals told me, those who could afford it started buying water to bathe in, lest they also develop skin conditions from the smelly water coming out of their pipes. The aquifer was dropping precipitously as dye units sucked fresh water out of it.

In 1996, the Supreme Court of India ordered dyeing units to either stop polluting or shut down. Meanwhile, the Tirupur Exporters' Association and the Tamil Nadu government routed fresh water from a nearby town to serve the factories—the blackened water was interfering with their dyehouse operations.

In 2011, the Madras High Court (Madras is now called Chennai) instated an even stricter rule: dyehouses were not allowed to discharge any liquid effluent at all. Tirupur's industrialists were now tasked with doing something no one had ever done before: not just purifying their wastewater but also creating a zero-liquid-discharge (ZLD) system.

With financial help from the government, I was told, small units banded together to build shared effluent-treatment plants, while large factories built their own, recycling the purified wastewater back through the system. After the implementation of ZLD, the water that had been brought in for factories was freed up for regular Tirupur citizens to use. I showered in that water during my stay in Tirupur, and my skin didn't react.

This story gave me hope that with enough political will, we can make progress on these issues. And anyway, this book is not about pollution in the groundwater. As horrific as that is, many skilled journalists have reported on it. It's about what's *on* your clothes. I wanted to speak to garment workers whose exposure to fashion chemistry isn't through drinking water or contaminated vegetables but is somewhat similar to ours: touching the clothing fresh from the dye units, breathing in the fibers that are coated with chemicals.

When I put the word out that I was looking for someone to

guide me through a textile manufacturing hub, a human rights journalist named Sujatha Sivagnanam got in touch. She was from Coimbatore, a city an hour's drive from Tirupur; had lived and worked for years in Tirupur; and had a deep network of contacts there. That was the final push I needed to start looking up flights to the knitwear capital of India.

When I arrived on a warm spring evening in May 2022, fashion trade outlets were reporting that Tirupur's textile mills were planning a collective shutdown to protest the huge increase in cotton prices. The garment factories were reportedly considering changing their product mix. "Most of the global markets demand synthetic products and we have to meet the buyers' demand on this," officials had told the Indian newspaper the *Financial Express* just a month earlier. "We are working on product diversification." It sounds like they were learning the lesson that the American textile company Milliken had learned fifty years before: performance textiles are a better bet than regular old cotton.

Sujatha was on the phone our entire car ride to Tirupur, and she managed to secure us a visit to the home of a garment worker after a long workday.

Just a year younger than me at thirty-four years old, Leelavathi was plump, with a round face and a ready smile. Like the other four garment workers gathered in that spare but clean and bright room, she wore petite gold dangling earrings and a colorful saree. Other family members wandered in, checking on the dinner bubbling on the stove in the adjacent kitchen, which filled the air with the smell of spicy home cooking.

With Sujatha's help translating, I asked the group about health problems. One woman told us she has leg and back pain from sitting at a sewing machine all day. The one leg that doesn't push the treadle to power the machine goes numb, and her son gives her a massage each night to get the blood flowing again.

And then there is the fatigue. A typical shift stretches for twelve hours or longer, so factories can satisfy our rapacious appetite for cheap clothing. Combined with the commute and getting food on the table for their families, female garment workers can only get four or five hours of sleep a night.

A 2018 health survey in India reported that 83 percent of casual workers in rural nonfarm occupations lack health insurance, and factory owners can bypass a law mandating regular health checks for employees by keeping worker numbers below twenty, a local community health doctor told researchers, and rotating them through so they're never officially permanent.

The truth is, as several people rightly pointed out to me, many of their health problems can't be isolated from malnutrition, long work hours, lack of preventative care, and poor living conditions. Still, there's been plenty of research showing the kind of unique illnesses garment workers suffer from. Respiratory problems— including abnormal lung function, asthma, and congestion—are their most common complaint. A 2021 report by researchers in Tirupur described how the fine dust from the cotton power looms gets into the noses and lungs of these workers, leading to bronchitis and weight loss. Between their runny noses and the heat, having a mask on is untenable. "When we go to the government primary health centre [PHC] in the village, they have very specific medicines for power loom workers," a twenty-five-year-old male worker in the region told researchers.

Researchers in the United States have identified something even worse called flock worker's lung, a type of interstitial lung disease associated with workers in factories that create synthetic velvets with short fibers. There's evidence that flock worker's lung can increase the risk of lung cancer.

Sujatha and I spoke to a former garment worker and now union secretary, G. Sampath. (In Tamil Nadu, in defiance of the caste system, the standard is to list your family name's first initial, then your given name.) He told us that he developed chronic asthma during his time in a cotton cut-and-sew factory, where they make things like T-shirts and shorts, and he still has to stick his head outside for air whenever he sweeps his home. He also told us about the horrors of dyehouse workers, who are mostly male. In 2019, several had died when they had been forced to climb into underground dye-waste storage tanks and had suffocated on the fumes. A local activist told us his father, who was a dyehouse worker, had skin on his hands and forearms that was shiny and brittle from working with the dyes.

Like the dye in the groundwater, the pathos of the industry permeates Tirupur society. Two decades ago, a local novelist, Subrabharathi Manian, wrote a story about a dyehouse worker who falls sick with skin issues. His disgusted wife refuses to be intimate with him, so he rapes her. She commits suicide. It won Best Novel from the Tamil Nadu government in 1999.

It's not just dyehouse workers who suffer. Garment workers who operate the machines, research shows, also suffer from skin disease, cardiovascular problems, gastric pain, and diarrhea. They attribute their health problems to the chemical hazards of dust, smoke, mist, and fumes that float in the air of their workplaces.

When I asked the group of garment workers about skin problems, Leelavathi exclaimed in Tamil and showed me the scars pitting her arms. Then she pulled up her turquoise-and-gold polyester saree to show me her legs. I gasped—the blisters were still there. While her arms, which are uncovered by the wrapped saree, had improved immediately after she quit her sewing job, her legs were for some reason healing much more slowly. Maybe because they still brushed up against colorful polyester in the Indian heat, every single day?

Hidden in Plain Sight

In the past decade, some version of Tirupur's regulatory cleanup has been happening around the world. Greenpeace dropped its bombshell report in 2011, based on effluent testing outside a dyehouse and textile mill situated on two different river systems in China, which together supplied Western brands like Abercrombie & Fitch, Adidas, Calvin Klein, Converse, H&M, Lacoste, and Nike. Their sampling found hazardous, persistent, and hormone-disrupting chemicals, including nonylphenols (NPs) and perfluorinated chemicals (the PFAS class of chemicals* Graham Peaslee had been finding everywhere).

The next year, Greenpeace purchased 141 items of clothing from twenty different large fashion brands that had been manufactured in at least eighteen different countries. Testing of the items found high concentrations of phthalates and carcinogenic amines in some of the products, and NPEs were found in two-thirds of the garments, in concentrations ranging from 1 ppm to 45,000 ppm.

Spooked by Greenpeace's ongoing campaign, the global brands it had targeted decided to get together and do something about this problem. They formed ZDHC, short for Zero Discharge of Hazardous Chemicals. Almost forty of the world's largest fashion retailers, including Levi Strauss, Gap, ASOS, Adidas, Zara, JCPenney, Nike, and Target, eventually signed up, along with large chemical companies and textile manufacturers.

According to everyone I've talked to, ZDHC has moved the industry forward significantly. It published a list of chemicals that members agree not to use, called a manufacturing restricted substance list, or MRSL. That's good not just for workers and communities where clothing is made but for shoppers, too. If a chemical is not used at all during manufacture, then it probably won't show up on the final product.

"I do think that especially in the countries that don't have strong policies, that initiative is really helpful," Yiliqi, a scientist and expert on toxic chemistry in consumer products at the Natural Resources Defense Council, told me about ZDHC's work. (As an ethnic

---

*The Greenpeace report says "PFCs," but in the past few years the industry has switched to calling this class of chemicals PFAS, as a more precise and accurate term. You might still see some brands say they are "PFC-free," however.

Mongolian from China, Yiliqi has only one name.) "Although we as an advocacy NGO think that there is so much more they can do." For example, she thought the ZDHC would do a better job if it moved beyond banning individual types of PFAS to banning the entire category from use. (It moved to do so in the fall of 2022.)

ZDHC also created a program to test the effluent of manufacturers and certify those that are not putting these chemicals out into waterways. We visited one of these ZDHC partner dyehouses in Tirupur, which serves brands like H&M, Primark, and Walmart. It was located down a byzantine network of packed dirt roads that seemed wholly inadequate for delivery trucks; the first sign we saw for it had the Oeko-Tex and GOTS logos proudly painted by its front gate. We checked in with security and took in the impressive complex as a group of managers came out to greet us. The multistory pale blue cement buildings with neat turquoise trim hummed like a beehive, their internal machinery at full tilt.

Despite giving us a warm welcome with coffee and freshly fried Indian treats, the general manager was hesitant to speak to us. I assumed he didn't want to get in trouble with his brand clients, but later I was told he was more nervous about his fellow industrialists. If I said *his* factory was the best, it would make *them* look bad by comparison. Indian industrialists protect their own. But after some reassurances (and a recommendation from a fellow garment factory owner), he gave Sujatha and me a tour.

We started with the effluent treatment plant, which is located out in front of the complex in a place of pride, right behind a life-size Ganesh shrine. First, we walked through a small warehouse filled with rows of piping, where we had to shout above the roar of water pumped through the system. Outside, two huge round pools clarified the solids out, and a square tank five and a half meters deep churned like a particularly unappealing hot tub. It was aerating the chemical soup so that the aerobic bacteria could munch on the chemicals and break them down. Ninety-four percent of what leaves the dyehouse in pipes comes out the end of the system as pure water, which is pumped back through the dyehouse. There's also some sludge that is sent to a cement factory, and some salts that are either recycled or stored nearby.

They told me they're not sure what to do with those salts yet. And later that year, news broke that textile dyeing units in Tirupur and the effluent treatment plants that service them have accumulated "mountains of salt sludge" from ten years of processing wastewater . . . some sixty thousand metric tons of it. It seems that the technology exists to process it, but it would cost $73 per metric ton, or more than $4 million to go through all of it. Who would pay for that?

Just building this huge treatment plant doubled the price of construction for this dyehouse, and 25 percent of the price of the rolls of cloth it sells to garment factories goes toward running the water treatment system. Nobody could (or would) make that kind of investment, I mused to Sujatha, unless they were forced to. She agreed.

Next, we walked through the dyeing and finishing process. It's way more intense than your typical backyard tie-dye project. My tour guides told us the raw, off-white cotton fabric we saw sitting in large rolling bins in the hallway had arrived chemical-free, the processing chemicals used in weaving it—such as sizing chemicals that strengthen the threads for weaving, lubricants, solvents, and binders—already stripped off at the mill (ideally, anyway). But it has to be pretreated again with all manner of substances: surfactants to help the dye penetrate the fabric, bases for cleaning the fabric, and bleaches to prepare it for dyeing.

In one room, there was an automatic dispensing system with large, labeled tanks—*hydrogen peroxide, invadine, puronal AR Liq*, and more—with pipes running down into the floor and then up into the shiny cylindrical washing drums in the airplane hangar–size warehouse. This state-of-the-art, computer-operated autodose system ensures that workers never have to touch the hazardous chemicals. In one room where powder dyes from well-respected global companies like DyStar are stored, we encountered a surprised worker sheathed head to toe in gloves and an apron, his curly black hair peeking out over his large goggles.

The safety data sheets (SDSs) from the chemical manufacturers are kept in a database where any employee can look them up. They don't contain the exact chemical composition, just the general components ("surfactants," for example) and safe handling instructions.

In fact, *nobody* but the chemical manufacturers knows exactly what is in most of these dyes and branded products. It's regarded as a proprietary secret. Chemical companies know that if they reveal the exact ingredient list in something they've spent years and hundreds of thousands of dollars developing, dyehouses or fashion brands can take that to another manufacturer and ask them to make the same chemical product, but cheaper. So even the dyehouses using the barrels of chemical products, and the fashion brands selling raincoats and underwear coated with these chemical products, usually don't know what's inside them.

Brands have started getting testy about this information hole. Earlier in 2022, a small group of organizations and companies— H&M, Nudie Jeans, Tarkett floor and wall coverings, Shaw carpeting, Seventh Generation cleaning products—sent an open letter calling for the European Commission to "examine how to best incentivize chemical suppliers to share full information on chemical content and hazardous properties."

"Even for us influential, large, and multinational brands, it is challenging and often impossible to receive sufficient and relevant information from suppliers on the chemical content. We can only assume that this is even more difficult for [small and medium-size companies]," the letter said.

So, fashion brands tell chemical companies and dyehouses what they *don't* want in there. That's the manufacturing restricted substance list that ZDHC has come up with. And then, if they feel like it and think it's worth it to spend the money, brands have fashion items tested. The factory we were touring sends their products once a year to Oeko-Tex to be tested for hazardous substances, and they receive a certificate in return. They buy certified chemical products from reputable suppliers and even test the products themselves to ensure they aren't hazardous. When I asked the manager if there were colors they couldn't get in certified form, he said peacock blue was out, but the brand designers they work with are always happy to find an alternative.

But there are gaps in this system. The next month on a video call, Ali Abdullah, the founder and managing director at Diamond Denim by the Sapphire Group in Pakistan, told me a story about the time his factory shipped an order of jeans to a brand in Europe. The brand did some testing and found restricted azo dye in the black polyester pockets.

"We traced it down to a supplier of the pocketing. He claimed that the supplier is Oeko-Tex certified, so there's no way that there can be azo in there," Abdullah said. "Three, four years we were buying from the supplier and we never had an issue. And then all of a sudden it comes up, most probably because they were trying to source cheaper chemicals." I asked him how that could have happened. "The way the system works for Oeko-Tex is that every year you send them a fabric to test. You're not testing each production." A dyehouse can secretly switch chemicals any time during that year to save money (even though they are supposed to resubmit a new sample for testing). "I have heard many instances of this happening," he said. (The jeans were incinerated, by the way, and Diamond Denim had to eat that cost. The supplier always loses in this game.)

The next step in this process is often printing. In the next room, we watched a huge bolt of pale pink fabric roll out, little black cartoon character outlines appearing on it on the other side. It looked like it would be made into children's clothing.

The workers moving around the printing machine didn't have respirators, just cloth masks like us. It smelled bad, like an extremely low-budget nail salon. (Fun fact: nail polish and fashion can both contain toluene.) The manager told me that they're looking for an alternative to the solvent required for printing, but so far, this is what they have to use. Another garment factory owner told me he tries to avoid printing if at all possible, because it's so hard to do it and have the final product pass the safe chemistry tests.

In the final step, fabric softeners are applied to the fabric to give it a nice hand feel. They will wash off within ten wears, the manager told us with a shrug. It's just so it feels nice in the store when you or I pick it up and try it on.

This is for a dyehouse that mainly works with cotton, by the way. At dyehouse that give synthetic performance fabrics moisture-management, stain-resistant, and waterproof technologies, the list of finishes and chemicals used is much, much longer: resins, ammonium compounds, silicones, polyurethanes, formaldehyde, and PFAS are a few. And they use those azo disperse dyes that the Duke researchers pointed out are, at the very least, skin sensitizers.

During our final factory visit, to an Indian athletic brand that does its own cut-and-sew in Tirupur, the owner told me there is a safer solution to giving synthetic fabric color: dope dying. This is when the color is put into the synthetic threads as they're created. Dope dying is actually a cheaper process, and because it doesn't require disperse dye, or water- and chemical-filled dye baths, it's seen as an environmentally superior process. But the drawback is that because it's done during the polyester production, instead of after in the dyehouse, factories require a much higher minimum of fabric to be purchased, so ultra-fast-fashion brands, with their tiny orders of whatever is trending on TikTok that day, couldn't order dope-dyed fabric.

The other drawback, the factory owner told me, showing me the poster of dye samples on the wall, is that you can't get a true black, only dark colors approaching black. (An American polyester executive later told me that wasn't true.)

The giant dyeing facility we visited is what best-in-class safe chemical management looks like, at least if you want a colorful cotton T-shirt. And I have to say, by the end of the tour, I was sufficiently impressed. Without actually trying it for a day, I can't say for sure that it's a good or desirable job. But to me, it looked like better working conditions than a typical Amazon warehouse.

But—and this is a huge *but*—this dyehouse is not necessarily the norm. According to a July 2021 report by Planet Tracker, a non-profit financial think tank, out of 230 wet processing facilities it surveyed, only 23 percent had a chemical management policy and only 13 percent said they were working toward zero hazardous waste discharge. The smaller the dyehouse, I observed during my week in Tirupur, the less likely it has the resources to dye responsibly.

And just in case there's any confusion, ZDHC is a voluntary industry group, though most global brands you've heard of have joined by this point. More important, according to a back-of-the-envelope calculation by the fashion tech accelerator Fashion for Good (the best calculation we have so far, unfortunately), even the world's two hundred biggest brands account for probably less than 10 percent of the sheer volume of fashion being manufactured and sold around the world (though ZDHC maintains that it does cover the majority of what people buy).

"There's definitely a long tail of places that we don't reach," Scott Echols, ZDHC's program manager, admitted to me. The big ZDHC member brands, "they have huge [chemical] teams. You could argue whether they're doing this for marketing or whether they really want to change things. Sure, there's a little bit of both. But the brands that are in the middle, or the brands that are just a brand in name only, and everything is licensed product—they just don't have the resources internally to focus on it. If there was either a carrot or a stick, to force them to spend the time that they should on it, obviously, they would."

A Three-Tier System

I'd probably visited one of the "best of the best" dyehouses. What are working conditions like in other dyehouses? It's not so easy to find out.

In Tirupur, as in many developing countries, there is a three-tier system for fashion manufacturers. At the top are facilities like the one we visited, which boast of their eco-credentials, have the latest efficient technology, cultivate a mutually respectful, long-term relationship with (mostly) European brands, and make a high-quality product, so they can charge a slight premium.

One step down are the export factories that work with American brands that don't seem to care about eco-certifications—they just want something that conforms with the bare minimum legal requirements. These brands are not above switching to another factory based on a few pennies' difference per garment, Echols told me, even if those pennies cover a wastewater treatment plant.

"Talk about giving the supplier no incentive," he said. "You give them a list of chemicals not to use, and they don't know whether you're going to be there next week, or next month, or next year. What really is their benefit, even if they use the right chemicals, do everything you're asking, but [you] say, *You know what, it's gonna cost a penny more a garment*, and walk away?"

Sujatha and I stopped by one of these more "price-conscious" dyehouses whose textiles end up in Western brands. Instead of having an airplane hangar–size facility, it had a smaller outdoor shed for the dyeing equipment, where the workers mix the chemicals and dyes by (gloved) hand. The dye process manager told us they buy their chemicals from Indian chemical companies or local traders. This can be a problem, because traders often source cheap chemicals as a by-product from other industries like mining or construction. And these products can be contaminated with heavy metals, phthalates, and halogenated solvents. If a brand doesn't require extensive testing of its products, these contaminants can slip through to store shelves.

When we asked the midlevel dyehouses whether the garment factory they supply ever sends products back because they failed a test, he said yes. But only for a pH imbalance.

Sujatha and I looked at each other when he said that. During our interview with the garment workers, the son of one told us he's a merchandiser for a garment factory. He works directly with brand production managers from large US brands, and many require them to have their products tested for a short list of restricted substances. The factory then emails the results in the form of a PDF to production managers, who give the go-ahead to ship. These are the documents that Jaclyn received when she worked in production for New York–based fashion brands, affirming the clothing was free from carcinogenic azo dyes.

I had asked the factory merchandiser what happens if the product fails the test. "If it has something that will cause problems to the consumer's skin, it's marked as failed and we cannot ship it. But, for other things, we can have the results changed," he told me. In other words, certificates can be faked, especially for things like heavy metals and phthalates, which consumers won't notice. But a pH imbalance will cause immediate skin problems.

That is why this midlevel dyehouses only ever has to fix pH imbalances. The rest can be hidden from brands, especially if the brands really care only about price.

At the bottom of this system are factories that produce for the lower-price domestic Indian market. These small dyehouses, I was told by several people while in Tirupur, use whatever the cheapest chemicals are, never test them or the products for safety, don't provide protective equipment to employees, and are rumored to dump effluent into the river under the cover of night and during the rainy season. In Bangladesh, where thousands of factories produce clothing to sell to their fellow 165 million citizens, factories use the cheapest and brightest dyes available, which often are restricted azo dyes. There is no regulation to make them do otherwise.

We did not visit one of the dyehouses for domestic brands in Tirupur, but a water treatment engineer showed us a picture of what he said was one. A retaining wall for the wastewater tank had given out, and its contents had carved a small creek bed into the soil. Now all that was left was dried sludge. He told us the dyehouse had gotten the seal of approval from the government pollution control board not long before this happened.

Later, I found in a *Newsweek* article a similar story. "In February 2015, a wall in a pit holding tannery effluent collapsed, drowning 10 employees in toxic sludge. The plant had been approved by two [Tamil Nadu Pollution Control Board] inspectors, who were arrested and jailed for allegedly receiving a bribe of more than $3,000 to approve the factory's license." I suspect the water treatment engineer was using a picture of that tragedy to support the sales of his own dyehouse-specific equipment. If so, the reality was even more horrifying than his fiction.

Several sources told us that dyehouses in the same area have drilled deep boreholes on their property and dumped sludge and effluent into them. From there, plumes of chemicals further contaminate the groundwater. Of course, the industry denies this is happening, and we're not able to prove otherwise. But we do know that the region's waters are still suffering. In 2016, a local newspaper said the government policy had failed to stem the flow of pollution, citing the still-dirty Noyyal River, the "salty and dark" groundwater nearby, the dead soil that stretched for kilometers on either side of the river and that could no longer support the diverse crops traditional to the region. And as recently as 2020, a local researcher called Tirupur "an environmental dark spot," saying the river still had foam floating on its surface and the farms in the area still can't be cultivated.

And yet, the government did seem to be making efforts to

enforce the directive. Just a couple of months before my visit, it had cut power to a dyeing unit in nearby Erode when officials found effluent flowing into an open drain. Similar scuffles had broken out recently in the state of Gujarat, in northwest India.

As Sujatha and I drove away from one of the dyehouses, I told her that a similar story had played out before in America, in an area on the Jersey Shore called Toms River. A book by the same name by the environmental journalist Dan Fagin describes how the Swiss chemical company Ciba-Geigy (now the pharmaceutical company Novartis) had dumped dye manufacturing waste in holes on the grounds of its factory complex for decades, starting in the 1950s, contaminating the nearby stream and the groundwater. Then, under pressure, Ciba-Geigy built a pipe out to the ocean so it could pump its effluent straight out to sea. That's exactly what a chemical manufacturer in Gujarat is building right now, and with the blessing of the government!

Ciba-Geigy continued to pollute its surroundings until the 1980s, when the EPA started cracking down on chemical pollution and Ciba-Geigy closed up shop, citing labor expenses. Eventually, Ciba-Geigy, along with another chemical company whose products had been dumped outside of town, and the water company settled with the families of children who developed brain cancer, nervous system cancer, and leukemia (without admitting liability). But none of this information seemed to have crossed the ocean to Tirupur.

I told Sujatha that there are dozens of still-toxic waste sites all over the Eastern Seaboard of the US where dye manufacturers and textile mills used to be. They're now fenced off and posted with warning signs. Inside, expensive remediation wells have been running for decades, sucking in groundwater and purifying it. Often remediation involves simply scooping up all the contaminated soil and putting it in a lined landfill. And still, the fully remediated sites can't usually be farmed safely.

"Even if all the illegal dumping stopped today, and everyone was acting perfectly, the farmers wouldn't see the difference," I told Sujatha. "Somebody is going to have to tell them that their farmland isn't coming back. Not for generations, anyway."

"Okay," she said quietly, turning to look out the window at the idyllic-looking pond at the center of the manufacturing neighborhood we were leaving, a pond that I guessed was probably still full of pollutants and empty of life. I wanted to apologize for what I said to make her feel so bad, but I couldn't take back what was an unfortunate and difficult truth.

We're All Connected

Leelavathi experienced the contradictions of this tiered system directly. She went to work when she was a teenager, sewing cotton shirts for foreign brands in a relatively high-quality factory. The hours were long, but the modern sewing machines had exhaust systems that filtered the dust, so she didn't develop respiratory problems.

After seven years working in that factory, she got married and quit to have her two boys. When she was ready to go back to work, she decided to get a job at a factory for the domestic market. Without the international brands breathing down their necks, the hours at this factory were much better, so she could spend more time with her family.

But there was a trade-off. This factory had her sewing synthetic garments, with their azo disperse dyes. Since the garments were for Indian consumers, there was no testing before shipping. The factory also lacked air-conditioning. The heat made her sweat, and the fumes from the fabric, heated up by the old sewing machine, pricked her nose. That's when she started getting the blisters. She finally had to quit in late 2021. She hasn't worked since then— garment factories are pretty much the only game in town.

In a way, I was happy for her. Her doctor had believed her and given her sound advice, unlike with the stories of so many other women I had talked to. What would have happened to her body next if she had continued working there?

In so many conversations with researchers and experts, I heard that what the garment workers and their communities go through is a much bigger concern than consumer health. "The workers that are creating these things, they have bigger exposure," Echols told me in a typical conversation. "The communities where they're producing these things—they're the ones that are facing the brunt of this. It's not necessarily the consumer. Yes, there's going to be situations of allergies, and you know, there's the potential for exposure to things that we want to get rid of. That solvent, by the time it gets to the consumer, yeah, there may be a little residual, and sometimes you can smell stuff depending on how things were treated. But the real exposure is when they pull that roll of fabric in the factory, and it's being aired out extensively for the first time. We're worried about a tenth of a part per million of something remaining. And yet we're not necessarily thinking about, well, what about the person that actually makes that chemical?"

Months later, when I was catching up with Claudia Miller, the TILT researcher, she shared that her team had done some preliminary research into the varying prevalence of chemical intolerance in Italy, India, Japan, Mexico, and the United States. She asked me to guess which country appears to have the highest prevalence. I guessed India, and I was right.

That's why I was here, in Tirupur, to bear witness to what garment workers experience. But to my mind, this wasn't an either-or proposition. Either we focus fully on production *or* we center the concerns of privileged Western consumers?

No. What I was learning is that, especially when it comes to chemistry, we're all connected. And I mean that literally, not in a woo-woo way. What goes in at the front end at these wet processing facilities not only gets dumped out the back of dyehouses, it can end up in our closets, on our skin, and in our own washing machines.

Many Americans comfort themselves with the notion that what happens in India (and Bangladesh, and China) is unfortunate but has nothing to do with them. But that's not so. The garment workers in Tirupur and shoppers in America may be thousands of miles away from each other, but we are blood sisters. We have the same toxic chemistry, from the same articles of clothing, in our same blood.

And it is doing the same type of damage to all of us.

CHAPTER 9

TRUST BUT VERIFY

The Profitable Industry of Testing Your Clothes

One hot August day, I got in my car in Brooklyn and drove to New Jersey, to the Newark airport, which serves the tristate area of New York, New Jersey, and Connecticut. But instead of taking the exit for the passenger terminals, I took an exit cryptically labeled "North Area/South Area" and found myself on a road bordering air cargo. On the other side of the chain-link fence, UPS and United Cargo planes were parked outside hangars, ready to take on their next payload.

I took a few more loop-de-loop exits and joined a caravan of big rigs, shipping containers from Maersk and Evergreen rattling on their trailers. They belched black smoke, their diesel engines roaring all around me as they menaced my little car. I was now in the marine port area, and walls of shipping containers in mustard, forest green, fuchsia, and navy rose up on either side of the road.

I managed to take a left turn into a parking lot without getting run over by an impatient trucker, parked, and was greeted by a muscular man in cargo pants and a short-sleeve Customs and Border Protection shirt. This was Anthony Bucci, the public affairs specialist who would take me on my tour of the Newark marine port and airport and show me what the US does to stop dangerous consumer goods from entering the country.

Neatly shaved, Bucci had curly salt-and-pepper hair to his shoulders, a result, he quickly explained in his second-generation Italian / New Jersey accent, of barbershops being closed during the pandemic. A former air force major, he hadn't even known what his hair looked like long prior to 2020. But his wife liked it, so he kept it, even though his fellow officers were giving him a hard time. I liked him immediately.

He led me through the CBP field office and upstairs, where he introduced me to Assistant Port Director Ed Fox, a compact man with gray hair, and Deputy Chief Lucille Cirillo, a straight-backed woman with dark hair who looked like she could pick me up and bench-press me.

Outside the office in the hallway, a map showed the vast domain of the New York / Newark port, from the Mid-Hudson Bridge ninety miles north at Poughkeepsie, all the way down to Manasquan Inlet, fifty miles south in New Jersey, west to the Delaware Water Gap, and east to the tip of Long Island. Except for the cargo planes landing at JFK (which is its own port) and a couple of private airports, every commercial shipment that comes by air or sea to this huge, bustling area is overseen by this office.

Newark is the fifth-busiest airport in the country, and second-busiest seaport after Los Angeles. "We think they cheat a little bit because they combine Los Angeles and Long Beach," Fox said. "We're busier than either one of them individually."

From the front of the CBP port office, if you look east toward Newark Bay, you can see the marine port, bristling with candy-striped cranes unloading containers from the towering ships, and orange gantries with cranes on top darting around, stacking and unstacking the containers until the correct truck or train shows up to take them away. Ten to twenty ships arrive here per day, the largest of which can carry sixteen thousand containers, some of which are off-loaded and new ones loaded before the ship leaves for its next stop. Around twelve thousand containers per day flow through all six marine ports under the purview of this Customs office.

If you look south, you can see airplanes floating down from the sky to land at Newark Airport. This is the largest US port that combines air and sea, which was useful for me, since I wanted to see how the process for handling those differed—what with the rise of online shopping and all.

Earlier that year, I had submitted a Freedom of Information Act request to the Consumer Product Safety Commission, asking for information on all the chemical tests it had done on shipments of fashion products going back to 2012. It was a big request, but I wanted to understand what, if anything, the CPSC was doing to protect Americans from toxic products.

The two federal employees tasked with finding me the information were nothing but kind and helpful, even if it took them about three months to finally get me the spreadsheet, which had more than fifty-seven hundred entries. (They also withheld the names of the brands that had their products tested—as the representative told me on the phone, they would have had to notify every single brand and wait for a response before giving me the data, which seemed unlikely to go well, and didn't seem worth the trouble.)

According to the document I downloaded, the CPSC, with help from the port officers at Customs and Border Protection, tests a fashion shipment on average every couple of days. Not bad, until you think about the fact that the United States' nine largest ports got more than 138,000 shipping containers of goods *per day* in 2021, and the US as a whole imported the equivalent of 94 billion square meters of apparel a year. According to the data I got from the CPSC, out of the 3,462 shipments tested over a decade, they seized a third.

Here's how it works. Seventy-two hours before the ship arrives, Customs receives a manifest listing all the containers and their contents, and they cross-check it against their database, looking for clues that it might have some sort of contraband. Most shipments are just fine, sailing through the radiation detector (to check for dirty bombs) and heading off to a store near you. But if Customs has a suspicion, or a request from another federal agency like the CPSC to take a closer look, the shipping container gets sidelined and taken to a warehouse, officially called a Centralized Examination Station. There, a mobile X-ray drives down the row of containers, scanning them to look for anomalies. Then they're unloaded into the warehouse for a closer look.

Customs officers don't do the unloading themselves—the warehouse staff does. When I asked them about hazardous fumes coming out of the shipping containers, they all said it hadn't happened in recent memory. But in other countries such as New Zealand and the Netherlands, shipping containers have shown up treated with dangerous fumigants such as ethylene oxide and methyl bromide, the latter of which has been known to send workers at other ports to the hospital with seizures. The containers can also have products such as plastic that off-gas formaldehyde, benzene, toluene, and other carcinogens at levels above government workplace standards. A 2017 Swedish study called out shoes in particular, with one container having 1,2-Dichloroethane at thirty times the occupational exposure limits, and benzene at seventeen times the limits. Previous studies had also identified shoes as high-risk products, which tracked with what Dr. Ann McCampbell had told me about people with chemical intolerance and sneakers.

After the Customs briefing, we all piled into two CBP cars and visited the Centralized Examination Station. It was surprisingly calm and quiet inside the cavernous warehouse, which in total is the size of six football fields. To our right, loading bays opened to the inside of shipping containers. In front of us, products were laid out on the concrete floor, neatly organized and stacked in long rectangles, exactly as they had been in their container. The day I visited, there were off-brand baby strollers (potentially hazardous), old beat-up cars and motorcycles (potentially stolen), commercial-size buckets of Tide laundry detergent with Vietnamese labels (either counterfeit or not approved for sale in the US), and bottles of off-brand shampoo that had exploded and were leaking their shimmery, sodium lauryl sulfate-filled contents all over the concrete floor.

The officers walked me over to a folding display table to show off some of the things they had prevented from coming into the country: a cotton polyester quilt connected to forced labor in China, counterfeit Starbucks-branded earbud chargers with lead paint, fake Air Jordans, a giant plastic lollipop with lead (in the stick, not the candy itself), a mattress that was tested for flammability and released, an unsafe horseback riding helmet, and a truly terrifying clown bong. A china cabinet held fake Gucci, Birkin, and Chanel bags, and fake perfumes.

Seeing the kinds of things on the table confirmed what I knew: the CPSC tests only children's products for toxic substances and looks for only three: lead, cadmium, and phthalates.

When I had scrolled down the CPSC document from 2012 to 2022, I saw the fashion companies falling in line. In the early to mid-2010s, failures were common, especially for lead, which showed up in levels as high as 6,000 ppm in kids' shoes and clothing. But by 2018, manufacturers seemed to have gotten their supply chains in order—lead was a rare contaminant. The downward trend showed what a policy with some teeth could do.

This was another thing I had confirmed in Tirupur at the garment worker's home. The merchandiser said the garment factory and testing lab don't attempt to mask failures on children's clothing for lead, cadmium, and phthalates. Having a shipment rejected at the ports would be a very expensive mistake.

"There's systems set up so that for every kids' garment, people figured out how to generate a certificate that showed that it met the requirements of CPSIA," Scott Echols, program director at the industry group ZDHC, told me. CPSIA is the Consumer Product Safety Improvement Act of 2008, which specifically targeted children's products. "But they weren't going to do that until there was actually legislation. There were brands that saw it as a need internally, but unless there's something pushing it, it just doesn't happen."

Once a shipment gets released into the wilds of America's stores, it's rare that it gets recalled. The list of CPSC's fashion recalls for a toxic chemical in the last decade is exceedingly short: a Primark nose piercing with elevated nickel in 2021, kids' winter boots sold by Zulily with lead in 2020, kids' sunglasses with lead, and Fitbit wristwatches because of *nine thousand* reports of allergic reactions in 2014. (That was still, somehow, a voluntary recall.) Oh, and Dr. Martens voluntarily initiated a recall of boots in 2017 because of benzidine in the tongue lining. (That's the chemical connected to cancer in dye factory workers.) That's about it.

That's not to say that there have been no reported problems with fashion products. The CPSC also has a handy website called Safer-Products.gov where you can peruse all the public reports of reactions. Going back only two years revealed that various consumers have complained about Shein jeans that caused sores that looked like ringworm; cheap jewelry that gave a woman hives all over her neck, ears, wrist, and fingers; moccasins and Skechers slip-ons that gave feet chemical burns; black $3.99 tights bought at the grocery store that made a woman ill for days; a Lane Bryant bra; Walmart sandals (several times); a flannel shirt; detergent; and dryer sheets.

Relistening to my interview with Echols, it struck me that he specifically talked about brands getting their *documents* in order. They had learned to play the bureaucratic game, but had they actually cleaned up their products?

A supervisory officer, Alexey, joined us and said in his mild Ukrainian accent that his officers had just found boxes of sweatshirts in a shipment that was supposed to be food. He walked us through the refrigerated section of the warehouse to show us the goods, telling me on the way that somewhere between 25 to 40 percent of his inspections are done because of a CPSC request.

In the chilly food section, we examined the boxes addressed to a bastardized spelling of Carlstadt, New Jersey. Inside, green fleece sweaters were embroidered with the logo of the Minnesota Wild hockey team. Clearly fakes.

Counterfeits are a huge deal at this port. Often, when the Consumer Product Safety Commission asks Customs to target a shipment, Customs has already flagged the same one. And yes, counterfeit toys and children's clothing are often dangerous. They're flammable, have a choking hazard, or are filled with lead. The Department of Homeland Security is also very interested in counterfeits because they're a good way to fund things like terrorism. Sure, drugs are profitable, but if you get caught, there will be hell to pay. The consequences for getting caught with a fake Gucci are relatively benign.

When I first talked to Bucci on the phone, he mentioned that he knew nothing about restricted chemicals. On-site, I kept pressing the officers on this core question: Do they pull and examine shipments of name-brand fashion products—not just counterfeits— for restricted substances? But they couldn't say. "You've got so much on your plate," I tried to clarify. "When I say those words to you, I'm just wondering if you're like, *Oh yeah, totally, like it's a lot of what we do* or if you're like, *Ah, we have a lot of other things that we're focused on.*"

They all jumped in. "We care. We care very much," Cirillo said.

"We have familiarity with and we have had interactions with issues with lead-based paint. We had those lead in the toothpaste," Fox added.

"We've had lead in handbags," Cirillo added. "And you know what? I have children. Yeah, I care about what my kids are buying off the shelves from, you know, some of these five-and-dime stores."

"Don't go to Canal Street," Fox said when I asked what advice they would give to regular people based on what they've seen.

"We have families, like Lucille is saying, we live in the community," Bucci said. "So we're doing as much as we can to protect not only our neighbors, but our own family."

I saw them all more clearly at that moment, not just as all-knowing federal officers, but as people: the children of immigrants, with their own children, trying to achieve the American dream and protect their fellow citizens from the poisoned products hidden in an overwhelming tide of *stuff.*

With the sheer volume of goods flowing through the port, they have to trust that "legitimate trade"—that is, products imported by large brands—meets all the legal requirements. They have enough on their hands as it is, catching shipments of cocaine, counterfeit goods, and stolen cars. "Let's say, 99.9 percent of the trade is legitimate; it's that 0.1 percent that we're looking for," Bucci said. "So we can't hold up the economic engine of the United States, but we have an enforcement responsibility."

The marine cargo warehouse was chill (and chilly, filled with delicious snacks on their way to Chinatown and Koreatown). But the process is a lot less leisurely for the air cargo examination facility. I couldn't visit that part, and there was nothing to see at lunchtime on a Wednesday anyway. There, officers work through the night to examine and release air cargo from FedEx and DHL, which have promised three-day delivery for things as unimportant as a pair of fuzzy socks. That warehouse has a lot less time to deal with what has become a deluge of slippery plastic polybags pouring through the airport.

Since 2016, when Congress raised the *de minimis* on shipments from $200 to $800, air shipments of small packages have exploded. Essentially, anything worth less than $800 doesn't go through the same process of Customs scrutiny and is not charged import duties. This has created a big loophole for ultra-fast-fashion brands to invade the US market, shipping five-dollar tops straight to customers. Imagine: you can fit eighty or more items from Shein into one box before it will undergo even the basic check that a shipping container filled with the same item would. "That means that they can bring things in without the same restrictions that they would have previously had," Fox said. "I think it makes it just a bit of a challenge for us; we need to alter the approach that we take to protect the public and make sure that we're able to ensure that e-commerce flourishes."

The pandemic exacerbated the problem by sending everyone online and into their Instagram feeds to shop. Even Bucci told me he bought some travel clothing off a Facebook ad before his big family trip to Italy earlier that year. It was garbage quality, of course. He donated the items to Goodwill without wearing them.

Later, Cirillo asked me, "So I'm just curious, what have *you* seen that *I* need to stay away from?"

I stammered a response, trying to summarize for this professional and mother what I'd learned. Honestly, I'd seen too much.

What Laws?

At this point, there might as well be a tag inside Lady Liberty's dress saying, "Give me your cheap, your toxic, your wrinkled fashion yearning to be worn, the wretched refuse of your crowded factories." That's because the United States, among developed countries, has a very lax attitude toward toxic chemicals—especially if they're on clothing and accessories.

"The general perception is there are laws against all these things," Scott Echols of the ZDHC told me. "Which there aren't."

Looking at the anemic list of the CPSC's tested and recalled products, it was clear to me that consumers are asking for protection, and not getting it. And I'm not the only one who has noticed that the CPSC is not exactly its best self these days. In June 2021, a large group of surprising bedfellows—including the American Apparel & Footwear Association, the American Chemistry Council, Breast Cancer Prevention Partners, Consumer Reports, Earthjustice, and the Natural Resources Defense Council—banded together to send a letter asking Congress to give the CPSC more money.

"The agency is significantly underfunded and therefore short staffed compared to other federal health and safety regulatory agencies," the letter said, pointing out that its budget is "by far the smallest among federal health and safety regulatory agencies," and it struggles to keep up with the work of overseeing fifteen thousand different types of consumer products. That the American Chemistry Council and Earthjustice could agree on anything was startling. The situation must be very bad.

I mean, we did start from a major disadvantage. The Toxic Substances Control Act of 1976 allowed in an estimated sixty-four thousand chemicals without ever having them tested, and the EPA has not attempted to fully ban a chemical since the 1980s. Asbestos, for example, is still technically allowed to be used in some factories, and to be in some consumer products. Because there is a clearly proven link between asbestos and mesothelioma, and companies fear paying out expensive settlements, it's disappeared from store shelves.

For fashion chemistry, we may never get to the point where you can link cancer or infertility to the use of PFAS or azo dyes on clothing. So personal lawsuits probably won't save us here.

Even after President Barack Obama signed legislation directing the EPA to examine these permitted chemicals, not much has functionally changed. The EPA has been increasingly followed by accusations of collusion with the chemical industry. In 2021, whistleblowers from the EPA's New Chemicals Division, which is tasked with evaluating new chemicals proposed for commerce from chemical companies, accused other staff and managers of genuflecting to the chemical industry and rushing through approvals, often by cherry-picking the chemical assessments to make chemicals look safer, according to an expose by *The Intercept*. In a follow-up internal survey that came out in early 2022, EPA staff described the agency's work culture as "toxic," "extremely toxic," and "incredibly toxic." They meant that as a metaphor, but the irony wasn't lost on me.

One anonymous employee wrote, "When I joined the [New Chemicals Division], my expectation was very high because I was standing in the core sector to protect the American public and environment. But now I am failing all my excitement for the EPA, my duties, environmental justice for the public, and even as a human being."

The Problem with "Reasonable Risk"

At the base of this controversy is the battle over the *risk* versus *hazard* approach to chemical safety. Hazard is the inherent danger of a chemical. Risk is the combination of how dangerous a chemical is and how high your potential exposure is.

For example, we've learned that pure mercury is incredibly toxic. Ingesting it can kill you, if not seriously impair your faculties. A hazard-based approach would ban all consumer products containing mercury. But a risk-based approach says that you're fine to use mercury in a thermometer, as long as the thermometer is well made and kept out of reach of children. Sounds reasonable, right?

There's a problem with measuring risk, though, when it comes to chemicals in clothing. Far from being safely encased in an unbreakable container, chemicals are often held loosely on clothing. They come off in the air, in the wash, and on your skin.

"We know that chemicals are continually lost from any material over time," Professor Miriam Diamond at the University of Toronto told me. She and her students have been trying to model this transfer by looking through all the latest research, but there's not much out there. "It's a physical reality that the chemicals migrate to your skin from your clothing, with and without sweat. And that is accelerated when this clothing is skintight, when there's no air barrier. Even more when you're sitting on something, because you're pressing the fabric right against your skin." (When she said that, I thought about how I always break out on my butt when I fail to get out of my yoga leggings after a workout and flop down on the couch with my phone instead.) "Or how about when you're sleeping, and you're in a sleeping envelope that keeps whatever chemical is on your clothing contained. You're exposed when your clothing degases because you inhale. And finally you're exposed when you inhale the tiny fibers coming off your clothing."

There are a lot of unknowns, and industry folks leverage that blank space to urge us to not be too hasty in banning these toxic chemicals completely from clothing.

The US government's approach is to also consider, on top of risk, the economic impacts on companies making and selling this stuff. That's essentially what the American Apparel & Footwear Association cited when the New York state legislature proposed banning the use of PFAS—that class of stain- and waterproofing chemicals that are so persistent and toxic—in "common apparel" (i.e., shirts, pants, leisurewear, underwear, and other clothing not made for uniforms or extreme outdoor conditions) by the end of 2023. The industry cried foul, saying they would need until 2027. Again, this is for things like blouses and bras—we're not talking equipment for Mount Everest base camp.

Europe, on the other hand, is starting to get things under control. In 2007, the European Union put into place REACH (registration, evaluation, authorization and restriction of chemicals), which places the responsibility of figuring out health risks on chemical manufacturers and importers (instead of on consumers and overworked bureaucrats). It requires companies to register in a central database the health effects of any chemical product they create or import in amounts over a metric ton.

REACH has been a success; even employees of European chemical companies told me so. For example, it reduced industrial emissions of dioxins, furans, and PCBs by 80 percent in just seven years.

EU officials also realized that toxic chemicals were sneaking into the continent by way of consumer products. So now, companies have to disclose the presence of "chemicals of concern" in consumer products to everyone down the supply chain, including stores, if a chemical is at a concentration of more than 0.1 percent of the total product. Consumers also have the right to ask if there are any "chemicals of very high concern" in a consumer product and get an answer within forty-five days.

In 2018, the EU set its sights specifically on textile products, proposing and then following through on restrictions for thirty-three chemicals it classifies as carcinogenic, mutagenic, or reproductive toxic (what they call CMR chemicals). It included the heavy metals cadmium, chromium, arsenic, lead, benzene, formaldehyde, phthalates, azo dyes and their associated aryl amines, and quinoline dyes.

The EU now issues recalls or destroys incoming fashion products every week. When I checked its public toxic product notices in May 2020, I found fluffy baby shoes with excessive hexavalent chromium, a red feather-encrusted sweater containing restricted azo dyes, and a pair of blue-and-yellow flip-flops that had a panoply of chemicals: chlorinated paraffins, lead, and three different kinds of phthalates. Most of these were from cheap little brands, but the EU has recalled sunglasses by Bvlgari, Burberry, and Calvin Klein for excessive nickel; Under Armour face masks for containing a suspected carcinogen; and a Scotch & Soda suede jacket for excessive chromium.

Many companies still flout the rules, though. In 2021, the European Chemical Agency (ECHA) tested nearly six thousand consumer products for sale online and found that 78 percent were noncompliant with REACH, including jewelry with cadmium and children's toys with phthalates.

That's the stuff coming into a region that actually prohibits toxic clothing and tests for it. What do you think is showing up at the docks and international airports in the United States?

Well, we can get a sense by looking at California.

California's Prop 65 legislation requires brands to put a warning label on any product containing toxic chemicals like formaldehyde, lead, cadmium, some phthalates, and BPA. If someone discovers through testing that a product contains one of these substances, yet it doesn't come with a label saying it's carcinogenic or reproductive toxic, they can file a notice with California and then sue.

In spring 2022 alone, notices were filed against the retailers Five Below, Target, Ross Stores, Revolve, Nordstrom, Walmart, Burlington, T.J.Maxx, Jo-Ann, Amazon, and Macy's—some of them a half dozen times—for selling items like kids' backpacks and umbrellas containing endocrine-disrupting phthalates. Steve Madden and Vera Bradley were also dinged for selling products with phthalates. Ironically, they were found in Fjallraven's "eco" travel backpack.

"One of the things people often forget about Prop 65 is that it largely leads to reformulation," Howie Hirsch at Lexington Law Group told me. His firm, representing the Oakland-based consumer advocacy group Center for Environmental Health (CEH), sued and extracted two settlements, one in 2009 and the next in 2010, from almost one hundred retailers that sell in California, including Target, Kmart, Guess, Michael Kors, Calvin Klein, Forever 21, JCPenney, Kohl's, Kate Spade, Macy's, Saks Fifth Avenue, Victoria's Secret, and Walmart. The retailers agreed to get lead out of their products.

"Unfortunately, the most visible component of the law is the warnings. [They] can sometimes be useless and, you know, borderline silly," he says. But he compares Prop 65 to an iceberg. The labels are the tip poking out of the water. "Most of what happens as a result of Prop 65 happens underneath the surface."

Prop 65 has a few notable loopholes. A company has to have at least ten employees in California to be targeted. That exception was meant to avoid saddling tiny brands with such an expensive burden. But in the age of Shein and the ability of factories to by-pass retailers and advertise and ship straight to consumers, this loophole is a growing problem. These companies know that they won't be held legally or financially accountable for toxic products.

"We can't unfortunately drag a Chinese factory, for example, into California court to answer for their misdeeds," Hirsch said.

Up until recently, they couldn't drag Amazon into court, either. When Amazon was sued under Prop 65 for listing skin-lightening cream containing mercury from a third-party seller, a 2019 ruling supported its claim that it was more like Facebook than Target—it couldn't be held accountable for what other people were doing or saying or selling on its site. But in March 2022, an appeals court overturned that ruling, saying Amazon was in fact responsible for keeping consumers safe under California law.

"It took far too long to get here, but I do think that this is an important recognition of the realities of how we buy and sell products and consumers expectations," Danielle Fugere, president and chief counsel for corporate accountability nonprofit As You Sow, wrote in an amicus brief.

So Amazon might be forced to clean up its selection of *all* products, not just face creams or fashion. But it won't happen overnight. Even after the two big settlements a decade ago, CEH kept testing products and caught some brands continuing to sell toxic, unlabeled products. And keep in mind, Amazon is not only listing but shipping out product from third-party sellers. Its argument that it's not responsible for toxic products may be spurious, but it's unlikely that Instagram or TikTok will be sued under Prop 65 for what advertisers are selling on those platforms.

During our conversation, I asked Hirsch if he had any advice for me, since I wanted to have some of my own products tested.

"You know, if I were you, I'd be concerned," he said. "Testing is tricky. You could easily end up spending money and not finding anything."

Trust, and Occasionally Verify

My bookkeeper was confused. She emailed me, asking gently whether someone had hacked the PayPal account for EcoCult and gone on a shopping spree. There were a dozen purchases at brands she knew I would never shop at. "Don't worry," I responded. "It was me. I'm going to have them tested for toxins."

Not long after, a dear friend stopped by. We were catching up on the couch with glasses of white wine when she asked about my progress on this book. The pile of bags and boxes happened to be within arm's reach on the floor, so I started pulling them into my lap and opening them to pull out the neon and sparkly clothing and accessories.

"I mean, this is the detritus of our childhood mall experience," I said, brandishing the packaging. "Now they're all owned by holding companies and hedge funds. Those finance bros don't care. It's really sad."

"I think they got cool again, actually," she said, nodding at a shoebox with a nineties-era brand logo. "The coolest girl at my job would wear them." This was a high compliment—she used to attend Coachella and make best-dressed lists. I pulled out a pair of swirly American flag–colored rubber sandals. "Man, those are ugly," she laughed.

I next opened a package with Chinese lettering on the shipping label. It said it contained one vest, which was a lie. (A "mismanifest," Customs and Border Protection would call it.) It actually came with two sparkly tanks and two pleather miniskirts. I unzipped a polybag, inhaling the scent like I was checking for a dirty diaper. "Woof," I said, handing it to her. She smelled it. "Ugh, that's vinyl all right," she said, recoiling. She gently coughed, covering her mouth. "It's affecting me," she said. "I feel it in my chest. I'm getting phlegmy."

Then I remembered. When I had first told her I was writing a book about fashion chemistry, she had shared that she's sensitive to chemicals and can't be in places with scented products.

"I'm so sorry!" I cried, hastily gathering up all the bags, throwing them in the bedroom, and slamming the door.

"No, I should have known not to shove my nose in that bag. You don't react to that?" she asked, still coughing as I opened the windows and flicked on the fan.

"No, I don't," I said. "The research says, like, 20 percent of people have chemical sensitivity. That's not insignificant. But it's not everyone." I apologized again and again as her cough persisted over the next fifteen minutes. "No, it will pass," she said. And eventually it did.

I was surprised that my little experiment—buying an array of items that I guessed were the most toxic available from the most careless brands on the market—had already yielded results, purely by accident. But I wanted to be more scientific than that. I wanted to have them tested by the most respected lab in fashion chemistry, the same lab that tested the Alaska Airlines uniforms for Judith Anderson at the union. This label gave a clean bill of health and certification not only to replacement airline uniforms for American Airlines, Delta, and Alaska but to thousands of consumer goods you can buy at your local big-box store. It certified the giant dyehouse we visited in Tirupur, too.

Oeko-Tex was created twenty years ago by two European labs, Hohenstein and Testex, as Germany was moving to ban the use of certain azo dyes. It's an independent nonprofit that certifies brands, suppliers, and their products as safe. There are plenty of other players in this scene: bluesign, a Swiss company that provides chemical management training to brands and manufacturers; Global Organic Textile Standard (GOTS); Cradle to Cradle, which is all about clothing recyclability and biodegradability (it's hard to do either if something's got a toxic finish); and Scivera, which

screens all the ingredients in a chemical or fashion product to provide a full toxicology report to brands.

There are also at least twenty commercial labs that will test your
product for a fee. "And then there are consultants who don't necessarily do the testing, but interpret the testing," Hirsch at Lexington Law said. "So, you know, hired guns who do risk
assessments and miraculously never seem to find that there's any
problems with any of this."

Hirsch had warned me I might have trouble finding a lab that
would take my money. "As you can imagine, a lot of these labs
work for industry, and it's almost like a conflict of interest for them
to work for us."

"That's what I'm finding with the fashion industry in general,"
I said. "It is very, very, very, very hard to find a subject-matter expert who does not in some way work for the industry."

"Welcome to my world," he said.

He was right. Bureau Veritas told me they don't work with private citizens or media as a matter of policy. I didn't even try Inter-
tek, whose multistory building in Tirupur we drove past several
times.

Anyway, I was told that if I really wanted my test results to be
accepted as legit, the testing would have to be done by the Hohenstein lab to Oeko-Tex standards.

A thoroughly German organization, Oeko-Tex takes pride in
how strict its tests are—they go way beyond regulations in Europe
and the United States, testing for hundreds of substances. In some
of the tests, the material is dissolved completely into a solution and
the lab checks how much total of a substance is in there. In other
tests, the lab puts a material into a solution that mimics sweat, and
then tests the liquid to see how much of a hazardous chemical
leached out.

With twenty-one thousand clients, Oeko-Tex has massive reach
and brand recognition, even if most of the regular women I

interviewed had no idea how to pronounce it. ("Oh-koh tex" is fine.) Hundreds of thousands of components pass through these labs each year. You'll see Oeko-Tex labels on the websites of small start-up brands who were founded on an ethos of sustainability, as well as on sheets and towels sold at large retailers like Bed Bath & Beyond and Target.

Unfortunately, the call I arranged with an American representative for the German lab Hohenstein did not go as well as I had hoped. Far from being a nerd chemist (my people), he turned out to be a sales guy. He wanted to show me the entire presentation he gives to brands, and he got annoyed when I interrupted his languid explanation of how to use Oeko-Tex's website to find a material supplier with my pesky questions from the perspective of a shopper. (In my defense, I had only an hour and *a lot* of concerns.) More importantly, we seemed to disagree on some pretty basic assumptions, the most important one being PFAS.

I asked him how an Oeko-Tex-certified product like, say, Thinx period panties would have failed Graham Peaslee's test for PFAS. "They may be running tests trying to detect fluorine, but they're not saying how that fluorine was used," he said. He asserted that a lot of fluorine does not necessarily indicate PFAS. It is a pretty basic element, after all, added to toothpaste and drinking water as fluoride.

Later, I put this question to Miriam Diamond at the University of Toronto, and she did not agree. "I don't know who wears shingles as a fashion statement," she said. "But clothing does not have that level of inorganic fluorine. Fashion is not stuffed with minerals." While it could show up in makeup, which has minerals like mica to give it sparkle, there's only one likely reason for high levels of fluorine to be in fashion. In other words, if there is a lot of fluorine on a garment, more than 100 ppm, then it was intentionally put on there by a textile manufacturer. And that means it's PFAS.

I suggested to the Hohenstein representative that perhaps the panties contained the type of PFAS that the Oeko-Tex standard doesn't test for. There are, after all, more than twelve thousand types of PFAS identified by the EPA (so far—that number keeps going up). While not all of these are chemical products used on fashion—many are the result of others breaking down slightly in the environment, Oeko-Tex looks for only four dozen of them.

Earlier that year, I had discussed this with Joe Rinkevich, the founder of Scivera. His company provides brands like Nike with a full toxicology report on the chemical products used on their clothing and accessories. "Formulators are smart," he said. "They know the list just as well as Oeko-Tex does. And they will find a molecule that performs the exact same way as a restricted substance. It has the same carcinogenic properties or whatever the problem is."

But the Hohenstein rep stuck to his guns. He was throwing a lot of science at me, talking about carbon chains and saying that it's hard to come up with new types of perfluorinated chemicals. "That sounds super easy. But it's not," he said.

After our contentious call, I wasn't sure he would still want to help me with my little science project. But it turned out that as long as I promised to him, in writing, that I wouldn't name and shame any brands based on Hohenstein test failures, the company would assent to working with me. "We want to attract the brands; we don't want to shame them into working with us," he said.

I came up with my testing list by choosing brands that don't have a restricted substance list and aren't part of any of the organizations that encourage responsible chemistry. I added in a couple of slots for knockoffs and ultra-fast-fashion brands that seem to follow me around the internet with their low-quality banner ads. My goal was to buy products from brands that the average woman has easy access to, yet that don't seem to care one whit about their customers' health. And I was looking for high-risk products: T-shirts with printed lettering, neon colors, clear plastic, cheap jewelry, vegan and real leather products, and performance items that promised stain repellency. I bought a dozen items, some of them in twos so I would have enough material to test, and spent about $700 total.

One morning at home, I went through everything at our kitchen table. One mall-brand purchase came with a free-gift bag that had a musky, pungent smell that stung my nostrils and made me sneeze. When my husband saw me pull out a glitter robe and panties from an online store called SexyDresses.com, he gave me a stern look and said, "Do. Not. Shake. It." (He hates glitter.) After carefully unwrapping it, I found a tag saying it was made in Poland and stuffed it back in the box. It was made under Europe's REACH guidelines, so probably not worth testing. The long-sleeved surfing top had a smell that nauseated me. "Made in Cambodia," the tag said. "Keep away from fire."

The USC Trojans "100% cotton" shirt with gold foil lettering was made in El Salvador. I had leather gloves from a brand that was founded by a famous female designer but sold to a holding company in the early 2000s. It smelled like the interior of a car. A funky (the smell and the style) pair of translucent orange heels had a label that just said "all man-made materials." PVC? PU? Who knows! The boys' school uniform pants were made in Bangladesh and had an accidental poem on their tag: "Stain-resistant fabric makes spills bead up, roll off / Wrinkle resistant for a neat appearance / Still 100% cotton for comfort."

When I sent the list to the Hohenstein rep, he warned me, "I'm not sure of your budget, but this will not be inexpensive." He told me if I was on a budget, the first to go should be the sandals, surf top, boys' uniform pants, and the gloves—all from mass-market mall brands. He was pretty sure these brands were managing their chemicals well and the lab wouldn't find anything. I had found no indication that they were doing any chemical management, but I figured he knew something I didn't.

Over the next couple of weeks, he and I sent spreadsheets and emails back and forth, and I got on the phone with him to go over the proposed testing matrix. I had decided I wanted the free-gift bag tested, instead of the actual product I paid for. "Promo is always a problem," he agreed. He recommended I test for just a few classes of chemicals per item—things like formaldehyde, heavy metals, restricted dyes, and solvents. The Standard 100 certification would be far more comprehensive. But it could never test for every possible substance using its current methods. (Heather Stapleton and Lee Ferguson's mass spectrometry is apparently still too cutting edge for commercial labs. Or maybe too good.)

When he sent the final invoice, my jaw dropped. The total cost would be $17,000—forty-two times more than what I paid for all the products. And that was after I lopped a bunch of stuff off my wish list.

"If I were going to pare things down, I would always choose the things that have plastic," he said. "I can trim this down. I'll pick a couple of things I would drop." A few days later, he sent a new suggested testing matrix. Now it was at $13,000. I cut it down further and made myself a tiny, sad testing list.

> Free-gift-with-purchase drawstring bag from a mall
> brand: $1,288
> Red-and-white cotton, foil-print collegiate shirt from
> an online sports store: $2,163
> Neon-orange translucent heels from a mall brand:
> $2,242
> Pink faux-leather miniskirt from a large Chinese
> brand: $1,579
> Knockoff "Longchamp" bag I bought on Canal
> Street: $2,366
> Total: $9,638

I stared for a long time at the list and the numbers. Two months of New York City living expenses. It was ridiculous. Offensive. How could I possibly justify spending this much money? I stared at the list and the dollar signs some more. Would this provide me with the proof I needed to convince the experts, the brands, and you that the kind of fashion you can buy online and in stores is toxic?

According to Maxine Bédat's book *Unraveled: The Life and Death of a Garment*, the Swedish Chemicals Agency (KEMI) has identified twenty-four hundred textile-related substances and estimated that 10 percent of them are considered a potential risk to human health. This test would be looking for only half that, especially since I was going the "budget" route and testing only for a few classes of chemicals per item. So even if everything passed, it was no guarantee that it was all actually free of toxic chemicals. What if the pink vinyl skirt, the one that made my friend physically ill, came back with a clean bill of health because we didn't test for the right substances? It was a huge gamble.

Plus, there was already plenty of evidence that our clothing is toxic, with more and more tests coming out from nonprofits showing the vast array of restricted substances in all types of fashion.

And yet, I wanted to know how this works. Even if all I got from spending almost $10,000 was the insight that this system is laughably out of reach for normal people. I decided that this is what my book advance was for.

I wrote back, "Let's do it." The Hohenstein rep's assistant sent me the invoice, and, flinching, I wired the money.

But before I could make it to FedEx, the American Apparel & Footwear Association came out with a report that made my test of the fake Longchamp tote redundant. Out of forty-seven counterfeit products it had tested, seventeen failed for things like arsenic, lead, and phthalates. One product had six thousand times the limit of cadmium. I figured I didn't need more proof that knockoffs are toxic, so I took the faux Longchamp tote out and threw in the leather gloves, and shipped it all off to Germany.

Who Do You Believe?

"I am surprised how well the products performed," the Hohenstein representative wrote three weeks later, attaching a PDF. There were only two official failures. The USC shirt's foil print failed, with 6.8 ppm over the 10 ppm limit of pentylphenol, a type of alkylphenol that is persistent, bioaccumulative, and toxic. It's often used in paints and coatings. The gloves, which he had told me weren't worth testing, also failed with 335.9 ppm of chromium (III)—136 ppm over Oeko-Tex's limit—as well as .29 ppm of nickel and 41.8 ppm of the endocrine disruptor NPEO. My mind went back to Debbie in Gloversville.

The stinky free-gift bag didn't fail, but the lab did detect .2 ppm of nickel and .027 ppm of DEHP, a phthalate and endocrine disruptor. The also-stinky orange heels contained formaldehyde and two solvents: DMAc and DMF. Both are classified as reproductive toxins, and the Centers for Disease Control and Prevention (CDC) says that DMF can be absorbed through the skin and is toxic to the liver. Cancer has turned up in workers who were employed in factories with DMF fumes. The CDC also says, "DMF is known to increase the absorption of some substances." That is, it could interact with other toxic chemicals to make your exposure to it worse. The state of New Jersey's fact sheet on DMAc says, "High or repeated exposure can affect the brain, causing depression, hallucinations, and personality changes. It also may damage the liver." But both the substances were under the official limit. So the shoes passed.

The miniskirt that caused my friend's reaction turned up formaldehyde close to the limit, 9 ppm of antimony, .07 ppm of tetraethyltin, and .01 ppm of DMF. But it technically passed. My friend's body said one thing. The lab said another. Who would you believe?

"What do you think out of those substances would cause it to stink and then cause a reaction in my friend who smelled it?" I wrote to the Hohenstein representative. "I'm guessing the tetra-ethyltin, since I see on a hazard sheet it can cause breathing problems and the OSHA limit is .1 ppm over the course of the workday, right above what was in the skirt." (Repeated exposure to this organotin can also cause brain damage.) I also asked how Oeko-Tex had come up with those limits.

He wrote back trying to calm me down, telling me that I shouldn't draw any conclusions from the detection of chemicals under the limit or try to figure out where a smell came from.

"Each and every limit established in ST100 (and other standards) are different—sometimes based on data showing a chemical is harmful or can be harmful to a person," he wrote. "Sometimes that is related to direct skin contact, sometimes inhalation, sometimes they can be based on non-human studies or even similarities to other molecules structurally."

Really, the limits that labs use to declare something is safe are often best guesses or just tradition. Almost all the research we have on chemicals comes from factories where employees' exposure to a chemical over a long period of time can be isolated, measured, and then compared to their rates of serious illness. That's how we know formaldehyde is linked to cancer: because workers in textile factories that had measurable formaldehyde fumes were shown to be more likely than the average American to develop leukemia.

But to my knowledge, there's no research on the health effects of wearing a garment with azo dyes, formaldehyde, PFAS, or really anything else that we know is toxic. There's no information or research on what might happen to my friend should she buy and wear that pink pleather miniskirt to go out dancing every weekend.

And what about the fact that all these chemicals are combined in each piece? I'm not speaking about cutting-edge science here. Rachel Carson, in her 1962 book *Silent Spring*, which led to the ban of the toxic pesticide DDT and the formation of the EPA, wrote, "A human being, unlike a laboratory animal living under rigidly controlled conditions, is never exposed to one chemical alone . . . Whether released into soil or water or a man's blood, these unrelated chemicals do not remain segregated; there are mysterious and unseen changes by which one alters the power of another for harm." She goes on to describe several gory examples of dangerous chemical combinations of "safe" products, or so they were considered at the time.

What's more, only recently did medical research tend to include female humans and animals—scientists feared female hormonal cycles would make the research results messy and skewed. As a result, some medicines have been found to be way too strong for women at what doctors were told was the appropriate dose.

At the same time, I was seeing in the news that Delta employees were saying that they were still having reactions to the new Oeko-Tex-certified uniforms. With the Oeko-Tex stamp of approval, more than ever, they were being labeled as crazy—or at least far too sensitive.

Seeing the results of my own garment tests, and understanding how a toxic overexposure can sensitize the body to tiny amounts of chemicals with a similar structure, I knew the attendants weren't crazy. They're just unlucky: genetics and their job had conspired to—in some of the worst cases—ruin their health, and their life.

Lying by Omissions

Just a week after I got my results, a report came out from the modern nonprofit Silent Spring Institute showing that 18 percent of the children's products it tested, including those labeled as stain resistant, water resistant, and even "nontoxic" and "eco-friendly," had PFAS. The brands included Lands' End, Gap, Old Navy, Children's Place, and Columbia.

That's when I realized that none of the items I had sent to the Hohenstein lab were tested for PFAS. Later that year in the fall, a study came out in *Environmental Science & Technology* with

Miriam Diamond and Graham Peaslee as two leading authors, in which they found that children's products—mainly school uniforms—marketed in the US and Canada as stain resistant had similar levels of PFAS to outdoor gear. The study estimated that on average, children wearing these stain-resistant school uniforms would be exposed to 1.03 parts per billion of PFAS per kilogram of their body weight per day through their skin.

Because I ultimately decided not to have them tested by Hohenstein, I guess I'm allowed to tell you that the stain-resistant, wrinkle-resistant boys' pants I bought were from Lands' End. The surf top was from Roxy, the sandals from Skechers, and I also got a purple bra from Lane Bryant. I can't say whether any of them have restricted substances, because I didn't have them tested.

I ruminated on the experience for weeks afterward. Why had the Hohenstein rep thrown the big mall brands out of the short list of items to test? He hadn't thought the gloves were risky at all, and they had failed spectacularly.

It finally occurred to me one night when I was trying to fall asleep that the Oeko-Tex certification, as strict as it is, ultimately benefits the *brands*. They're the ones forking over hundreds of thousands of dollars; they must get some value out of it. They want either to burnish their image as a conscientious and green company or to be protected from financial and legal culpability for toxic chemicals in their products—maybe both. If someone has a reaction to their clothing or finds a toxic substance, the brands can point to the Oeko-Tex seal—just like the Thinx CEO, Delta, and Lands' End did—and say, *That's just an individual sensitivity.* Or: *Our product passed the best test on the market.*

And yet, even with all its imperfections, Oeko-Tex is the best thing we have. And by "we" I mean those of us with the time, money, and education necessary to find safer fashion products. This is a privilege. After all, I was told that the reason none of my items were tested for PFAS was because that test is expensive, and I was on a budget. A tiny $10,000 budget.

"Sorry, it's not cheap for a company to have that work done. It makes it inaccessible to the brands that most people use," Joe Rinkevich of Scivera told me. Granted, Scivera could be considered a competitor to these other labels. But what he told me rang true. "It's not scalable. There's so many different items out there, to think that the world would go entirely to Oeko-Tex, bluesign, or maybe five or six other apparel-related eco labels—it's not possible. The average consumer . . . or let me take that back, not the average consumer. The person who buys Oeko-Tex-certified products, that helps them feel better about their purchase. But that's 0.1 percent of the garments on the market. And I know all those guys really well. Over the last twenty years, they've done great things for raising awareness about chemicals of concern in finished garments and inputs upstream. But at the same time, it creates almost a false sense of security. And if we really want to think of a solution that will make it safer for everyone, in this case, from a chemistry point of view, it's got to be a different paradigm."

If only all Americans had the right to know what is in their clothing and choose nontoxic alternatives! But all this testing is done behind the scenes, out of the view of the public, of researchers, of shoppers. If a product fails one of these voluntary tests, it may not get a certificate. But it is a private matter between the brand, the supplier, and the lab, protected by nondisclosure agreements and commercial relationships. That data or information will likely never make it out to the public domain, to governments, to consumers, or to researchers. And technically, there's nothing illegal about selling adult gloves with excessive chromium or a sweater made with red azo dye, in our land of liberty.

"You have an industry marking their own homework," says Emily Macintosh, policy officer for textiles at the European Environmental Bureau. "You have certification schemes and, potentially, a revolving door between the people writing the rules and people who are making money out of that same business model. If you don't make it mandatory for companies to act in a certain way, what we've seen is that action is not going to happen fast enough just on the goodwill of industry. I think if we have strong binding rules at the EU level or the global level, it's going to be much faster than waiting for the so-called frontliners, or the 'least-worst' actors, to pull the industry up."

PART V

HOW YOU CAN
PROTECT YOURSELF

CHAPTER 10

CLEANUP TIME

What All of Us Can Do for a
Cleaner Closet—and World

Whenever I reveal to a friend or acquaintance one of the many terrifying things I learned over the course of researching this book, the first thing they ask me is "So, what should I buy?"

So here you go: I'm going to share with you my expert tips on how to choose healthy clothing, shoes, and accessories—plus take care of them—so that you can protect yourself and your family from exposure to fashion's toxic chemicals.

Of course, this would be a much easier task if companies were compelled to get toxic chemicals out of their products and to give you the information you need to make safe purchasing decisions. But if you try to keep all these things in mind, you will clean up your home, reduce your and your family's chemical body burden, and even reduce the amount of toxic chemicals flowing into your local waterways from your washing machine.

It doesn't take a chemistry degree after all—just a bit of thought and care.

1. Avoid cheap knockoffs, unknown brands, and ultra-fast-fashion brands.

"I would say, as a consumer, if I'm buying from a global brand,

I'm not concerned," says Scott Echols of ZDHC. "I'd be concerned that the bag that I got on Canal Street would have phthalates in it."

Echols has a behind-the-scenes view of what goes on in fashion's supply chain. And he has a point. There are thousands of fashion "brands" out there with gibberish names that spring up to provide cheap knockoffs and dupes to shoppers. (Fun fact: Shein started out as a drop-shipping company with the gibberish name *SheInside*.)

This twenty-first-century strategy—manufacturing a product quickly at the factory after it is ordered and shipping it across the world—is called *drop-shipping*. You can tell a product is drop-shipped because it usually takes more than two weeks for it to finally arrive. (And it usually doesn't look much like the picture.)

I'm not talking about the small online marketplaces showcasing emerging designers, that let the designers do the shipping. I'm talking about borderline fraudulent brands that don't care about quality or their reputation because they don't need or have a reputation to protect. All they need to do is steal a few cute images from another brand or influencer and put them up somewhere you will see them, whether in banner ads or on Amazon, Instagram, Facebook, Poshmark, or other shoppable technology platforms. In September of 2022, for example, a brand called Kolan—which had been registered just two years earlier—had to recall two styles of children's footwear it had sold via Amazon because they contained dangerous levels of lead in the inner layer.

Because these manufacturers ship directly to the customer, there is no responsible entity such as a retailer or government body overseeing them. And because the size and cost of these packages are so small, they avoid the scrutiny that shipping containers get. These brands often won't respond to requests for a refund, nor can you take them to court if they sell you a dangerous product—because they are headquartered abroad and can easily disappear.

It's best for your health and your wallet if you avoid these brands altogether.

2. Find companies you can trust.

Many consumers believe if they just buy natural materials, they will be safe. But that's not necessarily so. A white cotton blouse can be processed with so many chemicals, like PFAS for stain repellency or an anti-wrinkle finish, that if you were to compost it in your backyard, it would poison your organic garden.

So you should look for brands that are fully committed to detoxifying their supply chain. These are not the norm, by the way. Out of the 250 largest fashion brands in the world, in 2021 only 32 percent had published a restricted substance list, and 27 percent had disclosed progress toward eliminating their use of hazardous chemicals.

Fortunately, you can find safer clothing from brands that are still well within the affordable range. In fact, many are considered fast fashion.

I hesitate to put names in print, because things can change from year to year, and even the best brands are not guaranteed to be 100 percent safe. But I *can* say that H&M, Nike, Levi's, Patagonia, and Eileen Fisher have been deeply engaged with chemical management for at least a decade. Yeah, I know: H&M! It's true.

This is not to say they are perfect, however. All these companies sell products made with synthetic fabrics dyed with disperse dyes, and Patagonia, as of 2022, still hadn't gotten PFAS out of all its products. But they have made more commitments and more progress than many other large, affordable brands you may recognize.

3. Look for third-party labels.

You can also check out the brands that have engaged in some of these organizations and partnerships around safe chemistry:

- **Afirm Group:** The brands that are a part of Afirm subscribe to a common product restricted substance list (RSL) and have some of their products tested for hazardous chemicals. You can find a list of brands that work with Afirm on its website: Afirm-Group.com.

- **bluesign:** Brands can source from bluesign-partnered facilities that use safe chemistry, or source bluesign-approved fabric. Look for the bluesign logo or name on fashion brand websites, either in the product description or on the "About" or "Sustainability" page.
- **GOTS:** This label audits factories to ensure they're using chemistry that is approved under organic principles. Look for the label on fashion brand websites, either in the product description or on the "About" or "Sustainability" page.
- **Oeko-Tex:** While I showed the potential loopholes of this label, it's still one of the best we have. It audits facilities for chemical safety and tests final products to ensure they are free from around three hundred hazardous substances. Look for the label on fashion brand websites, either in the product description or on the "About" or "Sustainability" page.
- **ZDHC:** These brands subscribe to a manufacturing restricted substance list (MRSL) and work with wet processing facilities that treat their wastewater. You can find a list of brand members at: RoadmapToZero.com.

There are other labs, certifications, consultancies, and industry groups. But these are some of the more well respected organizations when it comes to chemical management in fashion, and they are more transparent to shoppers like you and me. Keep in mind that they are all voluntary and unregulated, so they are not a guarantee that a product is completely nontoxic. Use them as a guideline or place to start your search.

And if a brand doesn't work with any of these organizations at all, I would avoid them.

4. Go for natural materials whenever possible.

Try to avoid anything that starts with *poly*—such as polyvinyl chloride (PVC), polyester, polyamide, or polyurethane (PU)—plus nylon, acrylic, glues, plasticky prints and coatings, glitter, and sequins if you can. These materials can either off-gas or shed toxic substances themselves, or very likely require sensitizing and toxic chemicals during the dyeing, finishing, and printing process.

Instead, look for cotton, silk, hemp, cashmere, linen, wool, alpaca, rayon, lyocell (Tencel), modal, and embellishments made with natural embroidery and glass beads. While I hesitate to recommend bamboo rayon because its production involves some seriously toxic chemicals, those chemicals are long, long gone by the time the final soft and safe product gets to you. And bamboo rayon is a fabric that many chemically intolerant people love. So if you want to try it out for your own sensitive skin, look for brands that have one of the labels I mentioned above.

5. Avoid "performance materials."

Performance attributes such as water repellency, stain repellency, wrinkle resistance, and easy-care fabrics are almost always achieved through toxic chemicals such as PFAS and coatings that can break down and come off the clothing into your house dust or onto your skin. I prefer to have a steamer and iron handy at home and take this particular task as an opportunity for catching up on podcasts or even just having some quiet, phone-free reflective time. (I even have a travel-size steamer/iron combo that I bring on trips.)

And I embrace the badge of honor from stains that come with heavy use of outdoor products like backpacks and jackets. If you really want to keep them clean and dry, you can use a PFAS-free stainproofing spray like Nikwax on your items.

Some outdoor brands such as Páramo, Didriksons, Vaude, Jack Wolfskin, Icebreaker, Keen, and Lundhags avoid using PFAS-based

performance coatings through a combination of physical engineering of textiles and water- and bio-based coatings. It is possible!

Also steer clear of anti-odor products, which are usually im-
pregnated with nanosilver, an unregulated substance that has been
making researchers very nervous when it comes to human and environmental toxicity. The EPA classifies silver as an environmental
hazard, due to its toxicity to aquatic plants and animals, and a
2005 study found that nanosilver is forty-five times more toxic
than normal silver. The research is still emerging, but there have
been studies indicating that nanosilver can be absorbed through
the skin, then distributed throughout the body to various organs,
where it is toxic. A study on oral exposure (nanosilver in food packaging) showed that it takes between two weeks and four months
to clear out of most of the body, but it can accumulate in organs
like the brain and testes, increasing the risk of damage over the
long term. No, we're not eating our clothing . . . unless you count
ingesting and breathing in the house dust that contains whatever
falls off our clothing, as we saw in chapter 2. Again, all this research is new—just like nanotechnology—and we need more. But
taken together, it doesn't make me want to sweat in anti-odor gym
gear.

Oh, and avoid permethrin-impregnated fashion products that
promise to deter insects, or permethrin spray. It's a pesticide that
you're wearing right next to your body—a risky proposition! Unless you're headed into an area with tropical diseases and you know
you're a mosquito magnet, it's better to create a physical barrier
against mosquitoes and ticks by wearing long sleeves, pants, and
socks with tightly woven fabric like linen and cotton.

6. Avoid supersaturated, ultrabright, or neon colors.

I hate to tell you to dress boring! If you love bright colors and
you don't have any skin issues, by all means, get yourself a fire-
engine-red silk dress or a hot pink cotton skirt.

But if you have sensitive skin, it could help to avoid neons, blues, and black, and instead look for white and cream, and muted, soft, earth-tone colors. Bonus if a brand uses natural and plant-based dyes! There are even some independent brands that source naturally-colored heritage cotton for socks and T-shirts from a farming outfit with a product called Foxfibre. It comes in pale brown, pink, and green.

Personally, I try to buy even my yoga leggings in at least 95 percent cotton. But if you absolutely require a synthetic product—maybe you're a big backpacker and need some lightweight hiking gear—look for white products that don't have any stain-resistant or water-repellent finishes. Evidence shows that the most toxic parts of synthetic materials are likely the dyes and finishes we put on them, not the material itself, and in its undyed state, polyester is shades of white.

You can also look for synthetic fabrics that are dope dyed, a.k.a. solution dyed. This means the pigment is incorporated right into the production of the synthetic fiber, which precludes the need for the sensitizing disperse dyes we discussed in chapter 2. Dope-dyed textiles are also more sustainable because they use less water and produce less wastewater, and they are less likely to release dye when you wear them. Patagonia, Gymshark, and Decathlon have all started switching some of their product lines to dope/solution dyeing.

7. Wash clothing with unscented laundry products before you wear it.

Some of the chemicals that are either intentionally added or that accidentally contaminate fashion during production and shipping—fungicides, biocides, pesticides, store fragrances, fabric softeners, dye that is *crocking* (coming off the fabric), and the like—will wash off if you throw the article of clothing in the laundry once or twice.

You never know where your new purchase has been, so don't risk it!

When you do throw your fashion into the washer, be sure to

avoid scented laundry detergents, dryer sheets, fabric softeners, and deodorizers, which leave a layer of toxic and sensitizing chemicals on your clothing.

A 2008 study from the University of Washington tested six top-selling scented laundry products and found that they all emitted at least one chemical regulated as hazardous under federal law, including acetone (the active ingredient in paint thinner and nail-polish remover), citrus-scented limonene, acetaldehyde, chloromethane, and 1,4-dioxane. And yet none of the chemicals were listed on the product labels. We can assume they were hidden as a trade secret inside the word "fragrance."

"Nearly 100 volatile organic compounds were emitted from these six products, and none were listed on any product label. Plus, five of the six products emitted one or more carcinogenic 'hazardous air pollutants,' which are considered by the Environmental Protection Agency to have no safe exposure level," the lead author, Anne Steinemann, said at the time. For her next study, in 2011, she showed that when consumers use popular scented laundry products in home washers and dryers, more than twenty-five volatile organic compounds can come out of the dryer vent, including the carcinogens acetaldehyde and benzene.

As if that weren't enough, mixing different scented laundry products can multiply your reaction. A 2002 study showed that when combined, allergenic fragrances had a *synergistic* instead of just *additive* effect on patients with eczema. You can think of *additive* like 5 + 5 = 10, while *synergistic* is 5 × 5 = 25.

Researchers layered two different fragrances on top of each other in a patch test and found that together they created an allergic response as if their dose were three to four times higher than what was actually used.

Buy unscented laundry products, and use wool dryer balls instead of dryer sheets if you feel the need. Personally, I've never used dryer sheets or fabric softeners in my adult life and haven't noticed the difference!

And don't use mothballs, which can contain naphthalene or paradichlorobenzene. Instead, put blocks of cedar in your drawers or use lavender sachets to protect your sweaters.

8. Don't dry-clean your clothing.

A typical dry-cleaning business uses a chemical called tetrachloroethene or perchloroethylene, commonly known as PERC. This chemical is so toxic that the EPA has required many former dry-cleaning sites to go through toxic remediation before anything else can be built on the land.

When you dry-clean your clothing or use stain-removing products that contain PERC, it can off-gas into the air of your home. PERC has been shown to affect the central nervous system, liver, kidneys, blood, and immune system and is suspected to affect the reproductive system.

Those "dry-clean only" labels? Those are often suggestions, not orders—brands like to put them on everything just to be safe. To avoid dry-cleaning, choose clothing that can be machine-washed. And definitely avoid a lot of fussy embellishments, especially if they are plastic.

If you do find yourself with these items, try to spot clean them and then hang them up to air out after you wear them. Hand-wash and air-dry your silk. Hand-wash your wool, cashmere, and alpaca items, and lay them out on a table to dry. Machine-wash your cotton and linen in cold water. While they can go in the dryer, hanging them up to air-dry will increase their life span and save you on energy bills. (I make an exception for towels: they are so lovely and fluffy after a good, hot tumble, I'll admit.) Some rayon or viscose can end up misshapen after a home wash, so if you have some, try hand-washing or using the delicate cycle, always with cold water.

If you must dry-clean, choose a "green" dry cleaner that uses liquid carbon dioxide. If you can't find one, take the plastic garment bag off your clothes and hang them outside your home in a

covered area such as a porch or garage to air out for a day or two
before you put them in your closet.

9. Buy secondhand or swap clothing.

Buying secondhand clothing from garage and yard sales, join-
ing a Buy Nothing group, or hosting swaps with your friends are
three super-affordable ways to get sustainable and nontoxic clothing that has already been washed several times and has off-gassed
its finishes. It's also a wonderful way to get to know your community. Just be aware that sometimes secondhand stores apply scented
products to their wares, and that scented detergent can linger for
quite a while on clothing that you've gotten secondhand.

10. Trust your nose.

If something smells like chemicals, don't risk it. Put it back in
the box and send it right back for a refund.

Keep in mind that these strategies are not fail-safes by themselves.
Because the fashion industry is so unregulated and opaque when
it comes to chemicals, you can absolutely buy natural textiles with
toxic finishes or products from more responsible brands that have
sensitizing disperse dyes or PFAS-based stain-repellency.

So now, I want to talk about what I want to see the *people in
charge* do.

You see, what I don't want to happen as a result of this book
is another movement that revolves around guilt-tripping women
about their purchasing choices. As much as I respect those who
buy organic food for their table, wooden toys for their kids, and
electric cars for their commute, I know that we cannot just shop
our way out of this problem.

As I've said many times before, it takes a lot of time, education,
money, and emotional energy to be a "good" shopper, especially
when the system is arrayed against you. It really is a privileged person

who can make the informed choices when it comes to fashion. And as we've seen throughout this book, even those women who have a steady income and a gut-deep knowledge that their body—or their children's bodies—cannot handle toxic fashion have struggled to overhaul their shopping and fashion habits. We can't expect everyone to hand-sew their own chemical-free, plant-based, certified-nontoxic underwear, as Karly did for her son in chapter 2. (Though you can certainly patronize her business!)

This movement for nontoxic should be inclusive. It should be about changing the system so that hazardous chemicals are not used on any clothing, shoes, or accessories, whether cheap or pricey, made in China or Europe, sold in India or America, meant for performance or for lounging, for children or for adults.

Everyone deserves safe fashion. And we deserve a global system that prioritizes our health above profit.

So here are the bold yet necessary changes I'm calling for:

1. Implement taxes and tariffs on untested chemicals to fund research.

There are somewhere between 40,000 and 350,000 chemical substances and polymers registered for use today. And the large majority of them have not been tested for safety. We need to clear this backlog. We also need to fill in our gaps of understanding when it comes to chemical interactions on clothing and in our bodies and the kind of exposure we get from wearing and touching fashion products that have toxic residues and finishes.

To pull this off, we will need many more millions of dollars poured into independent and university-based research institutes. To fund this, I suggest that governments heavily tax and tariff the sale and importation of understudied chemicals. I also would like to see tariffs imposed on fashion products that contain understudied chemical substances.

For an example of what this could achieve, consider the fact that Columbia Sportswear engages in what it calls "tariff engineering."

The company pairs designers with trade experts to guide their design decisions. For example, according to a *New York Times* story on the subject, "a water-resistant jacket triggers a 7.1 percent tariff, while a jacket that has not been waterproofed gets hit with a 27.7 percent tariff." As of the fall of 2022, Columbia has not yet indicated any intention of removing PFAS-based durable water-repellent finishes from its products. Perhaps because it likely would cost the brand money to do so!

Brands like Shein, meanwhile, locate their fulfillment warehouses right over the border in Mexico and Canada to avoid shipping anything into the United States that is worth more than $800. That's because any shipment worth less than $800 is considered "de minimis," or too small to be worth checking or levying import duties on. This encourages the production of ultracheap, toxic fashion—the United States reportedly gets more than two million de minimis shipments a day. China's de minimis limit is $7, or more than one hundred times less than ours.

As of 2022, Representative Earl Blumenauer of Oregon proposed legislation in Congress that would close this loophole.

2. Require chemical companies to register all chemicals in use and share any associated research.

As in Europe under REACH guidelines, chemical companies in the United States should be required to register information on all chemical substances and products manufactured and imported at amounts over one ton. And they should include in that registration all known health risks and research associated with each chemical and product.

Chemical companies should also be legally required to create analytical standards (lab-quality samples) of all chemical substances used in their products and send those to research institutes and government labs. A policy like this would have saved Kirsten Overdahl a year and a half of work had it been implemented before she started hand-purifying cans of textile dye. It could still save years of research—there are thousands more fashion chemicals to test.

3. Expand the Consumer Product Safety Commission's ability to test and recall toxic fashion.

As long as chemical safety is voluntary, there will be brands that prioritize profits over customer health. As we've seen, when the CPSC is endowed with even limited power to test children's products for hazardous substances, brands and factories make the effort to ensure these items are free of lead, cadmium, and phthalates.

Congress needs to expand the number of toxic substances the CPSC tests for, and they must apply testing to adult fashion as well as children's clothing. (I suggest starting with California's or the European Union's list of restricted substances.) There should be something pulled from fashion shipments for testing at every port—airports and marine—every day at the very least.

CPSC and port labs should use the PIGE test that Graham Peaslee uses to identify total fluorine in products, which would then indicate which ones need further testing, and the latest high-resolution mass spectrometry technology that we learned the researchers from Duke's Department of Integrated Toxicology and Environmental Health use to identify all the substances in a material. If CPSC labs had a full catalog of analytical standards provided by chemical companies (point 1), then it could easily identify everything in a product.

The CPSC also needs more power to force recalls of products that are toxic and sensitizing for consumers. Consumers who report reactions to the CPSC should have some assurance that their chemical burns are being taken seriously. They should be able to send in the offending article and have it tested by a lab that is not being paid by the brand that sold the product.

This would benefit not just Western consumers but consumers and workers in developing countries as well. The influence of this tighter border policy will stretch into production countries that fall outside the CPSC's jurisdiction. Because the best way to ensure that a product doesn't have a toxic substance on it is to not use it during production in the first place.

To pull this off, the CPSC needs way more funding. Everyone, even the chemical industry, seems to agree on that. Let's get on that, Congress.

4. Legislate all chemicals in classes instead of individually.

With at least forty thousand chemicals in circulation, even with all the funding in the world, it would be impossible for research labs to test every single chemical thoroughly to establish limits. As we've seen, once one chemical has been established as hazardous, the consumer product industry just switches to another similar chemical that is less studied and not regulated. We have tons of water bottles that say "BPA-free," but we don't know if they have another type of hormone-disrupting chemical such as BPS in them.

But we do know that classes of chemicals such as bisphenols, phthalates, and PFAS tend to carry similar hazardous properties.

"We're never going to be able to adequately study and test every single PFAS compound that is out there. It would take probably hundreds and hundreds of years to study all of them," Michael Schade of Toxic-Free Future told me. "If we say, *Let's regulate them one at a time*, millions of people around the world will continue to be exposed to potentially harmful levels of these extremely hazardous chemicals that are building up in our bodies."

Unless independent research proves that a particular chemical is safe, all chemicals with similar chemical structures should be treated as though they are identical to the most well studied and hazardous chemical in that class.

If BPA is banned in children's products, BPS should be, too. If DEHP is restricted, other types of phthalates should be, too. All PFAS, not just long-chain PFOA and PFOS, should be banned from production and use in consumer products. All azobenzene disperse dyes should be restricted, instead of just ones that re-searchers have proven cleave into carcinogenic amines.

And remember how the body's mast cells can start reacting to structurally similar chemicals? Who is to say banning one in a class of chemicals will do anything to relieve your textile allergy?

5. Ban the presence of endocrine disruptors in consumer products.

As I shared in chapter 5, scientists agree that there is no "safe" dose of endocrine disruptors. Because of the fertility and eco-logical crises caused by hormone-disrupting chemicals, and the health effects of even low doses, we need a total ban of endocrine-disrupting chemicals in consumer products, including on textile products and fashion accessories. That includes lead, mercury, ar-senic, phthalates, bisphenol A (BPA) and its cousins BPS and BPF, APEOs, and above all, PFAS.

6. Pass due diligence laws that hold fashion companies liable for pollution and worker health.

For too long, fashion brands and global suppliers have avoided taking responsibility for worker health by offshoring operations to countries with looser legislation and enforcement.

We have a good understanding of the health risks for workers of exposure to substances like formaldehyde, synthetic microfibers, and industrial bleaches. But many workers in countries like China and India continue to have unnecessary exposure when they are not provided proper training or protective gear. The communities around factories are poisoned by toxic effluent and sludge.

Much of the time this is due to brands demanding orders faster and cheaper. In order to make quota, for example, workers don't wear protective gear, which can slow them down. Or suppliers can't afford to invest in new equipment (like a water treatment plant) because brands won't pay any more for material made in a safe environment. And yet, when brands are made aware of the results of their sourcing policy, they say they didn't know and don't condone the behavior.

"The only way to solve it is to have a legislation that forces them to do something, or somehow takes the costs that they're pushing off—like the cost of polluting the waterway around the factory or health impacts on the workers—and include them in the triple-bottom-line costs, not just the cost per garment," says Scott Echols of ZDHC.

Several European countries, and more recently the European Union, have proposed due diligence legislation. Large fashion brands would be required to identify, then prevent, end, or mitigate the negative impacts of their business within their supply chain, even if the damage is outside the EU. This would include worker health and safety and environmental pollution.

For example, if a dyehouse worker died because he was told to climb into a dye-waste storage tank for cleaning, his family could hold the brands that had active orders with that dyehouse responsible. This would make brands think twice before walking away from a safe facility based on a slightly higher price. For example, brands would ensure that dyehouses in their supply chain have automatic storage-tank cleaning equipment that functions properly and might even provide loans or financing to factories that don't.

It's great that the European Union is pursuing this kind of legislation. It's time for the United States to do the same.

7. Go after greenwashers.

"Many companies for years have been saying, *We're getting out of the long-chain PFAS, no one is using them anymore,*" Michael Schade told me. But when his advocacy organization, Toxic-Free Future, tested water- and stain-resistant products for PFAS in early 2021 from Amazon, Bed Bath & Beyond, Costco, Dick's Sporting Goods, Kohl's, Macy's, REI, Target, Walmart, and TJX, owner of T.J.Maxx, Marshall's, and HomeGoods, they were surprised by what they found.

"The majority of PFAS-containing items tested positive for long-chain PFAS. And in some cases, they were the most abundant PFAS detected," he said. In other words, companies have been lying about the health and safety of their products, whether or not it was technically legal at the time.

Meanwhile, Gore-Tex has committed to eliminating what they call "PFCs of environmental concern." (As I noted before, some companies still use the term PFCs instead of PFAS.)

But that's redundant. "There's no PFASs that we believe are not of environmental concern, because the chemicals are fundamentally persistent," Schade said.

The Federal Trade Commission (FTC) has the power to penalize companies that make inaccurate sustainability claims on their products. It has fined retailers who market bamboo fabric as eco-friendly, since turning bamboo into soft rayon fabric requires the input of extremely hazardous chemicals (though these chemicals are long gone by the time it gets to consumers).

The FTC should do the same for brands that claim their products are nontoxic on the basis of certifications that test for only some hazardous substances. And it should go further to address deliberately confusing statements. For example, a brand should not be able to use confusing statements such as "BPA-free" if it hasn't tested for all types of bisphenol, or should not claim it uses a nontoxic durable water repellent in its rain gear if it's only just switched to other types of PFAS.

8. Require ingredient lists on fashion products.

The food industry, the cleaning product industry, and the beauty product industry all provide ingredient lists on their products, while staying profitable. In the construction materials business, architects, design professionals, contractors, and consumers can look up the health product declarations (HPDs) at www .HPD-Collaborative.org for over forty thousand building products for over eight hundred manufacturers. The information is not very consumer friendly, but it shows that this information can be provided even for performance textile products like synthetic carpeting.

"I have been talking since the early nineties about having disclosure of all chemicals that are in materials, goods, and products, including clothing," Åke Bergman, a Swedish environmental toxicologist, told me. "I don't understand that it is a proprietary right to not say what is being used for producing this product."

Consumers deserve to know what is in their fashion so that they can avoid substances that give them hives or a rash, or exacerbate their chronic illness. Every consumer fashion product should be legally required to carry a label or QR code that lists all known carcinogenic, mutagenic, reproductive toxic, bioaccumulative, persistent, allergenic, or sensitizing chemicals present.

"We are calling on retailers and brand owners to disclose chemical ingredients to consumers, including for articles like textiles," says Michael Schade, director of Toxic-Free Future's Mind the Store campaign. "If you're going to say, *Yes, as a business, we're going to regulate and restrict harmful chemicals in our supply chain*, you can't really do that if you don't know what's in the products that you're selling."

"It's not about putting the responsibility on consumers to change," says Emily Macintosh, policy officer for textiles at the European Environmental Bureau. "But it is about creating the kind of critical mass of pressure on companies that say, *We see you, we see what's happening*. This is not what people want when they buy something for a family member or for a loved one."

I've spoken to suppliers and chemical engineers about this, and they all say it is possible based on today's technology to list ingredients on the final product—as long as a brand doesn't switch from factory to factory, chasing cheap prices.

"Cradle to Cradle asks you to provide 100 percent transparency about the products if you want your product certified," Andrea Venier, managing director at the Italian chemical supplier

Officina+39, told me. "There it's protected by agreements and by law. So you make an agreement with the third-party companies. Everybody has responsibility amongst each other."

"I also want to see what's inside," said Kaan Şen, who at the time we talked was a chemical engineer and sustainability manager at the Blue Matters denim laundry in Turkey. (He is now a sustainability manager for Adidas.) "And the only way is legislation from the top."

If you agree with my plan of action, contact your representatives and ask them to reform the Toxic Substances Control Act (TSCA). Tell them which of the above actionable steps you would most like to happen. You can find your federal representatives at www.Gov Track.us/congress/members.

State representatives can also take action on your behalf, and a handful of states besides California, such as Maine and Washington, already have taken some steps toward detoxifying consumer products. Contact your state representative and let them know you would like to see action to protect your health from toxic textiles.

Maybe this seems like a lot. But I believe in the power of Americans to demand change. I especially believe in the power of women—the mothers and teachers, professors and researchers, designers and entrepreneurs—to demand that we care for each other and the next generation.

Remember that Earth Day was founded as a day of action in the wake of rivers on fire, toxic dumping, and the indiscriminate spraying of DDT and its effect on wildlife's babies. More recently in 2007, it was mothers in Canada who marched on the provincial legislature of Toronto, their toddlers strapped into strollers, demanding that BPA be restricted in things like baby bottles in Canada.

If we start tackling this as the interconnected and holistic problem it is, as a war against autoimmune disease, infertility, and chronic poisonings—instead of a series of disparate skirmishes over finishes, dyes, and plastics—I believe we can revolutionize our health, as well as start to reverse the environmental degradation of our planet perpetuated in the name of fashion. Hopefully, our children and grandchildren will look back on this time with appropriate wonder and horror about what we've been wearing.

CONCLUSION

I wish I had a story of vindication for you. A large settlement, an admission of the obvious truth. Some accountability by fashion and chemical companies. I don't. What I have is sadness, and anger.

By the spring of 2012, John at Alaska Airlines had no sick time left, and he was scheduled to fly two times a week. "What if anything can be done at this point? I'm at a loss for how to proceed," he wrote to Judith Anderson of the Association of Flight Attendants. He ended up in the emergency room that spring, and then again in July. In August he wrote, "I've had four instances where I have momentary lapses of memory; how long or how noticeable, I don't know. I find myself blanking out and snap right back and realize I wasn't there for a moment." He wrote that he had had difficulty breathing on a recent flight, but he didn't want to disrupt it by complaining. He was barely surviving on disability payments from California and then workers' compensation.

Alaska attendants reported to the union that their family members also had reactions after they washed the uniforms in their washing machines. Whatever the endocrine disruptors in the uniforms were, they seem to have started to affect the flight attendants' thyroids and in turn their hormones. Many attendants had irregular periods and debilitating fatigue. Some were losing their hair in chunks. Two women went completely bald.

Oregon Health & Science University offered to do a patch test for attendants, and Mary and John both went in. John's yielded nothing. Neither did Mary's, at first. But a week later, a burn developed on her skin. Her dermatologist saw it and confirmed that it was likely a delayed reaction and told her she should follow up. She called the doctor's office at OHSU, but the nurse who answered the phone noted in her file only that she wanted to have the results changed. It took six months for the burn to heal.

Anderson and the attendants had run out of organizations to turn to for help. "It made you powerless," Mary told me later. "You can't do anything. All I could do is hope that the union had more power to get the airline to admit that something was really wrong. And that never happened. They denied it all."

There was only one option left. In November 2012, a group of flight attendants filed a class action lawsuit in California against Twin Hill, asking for the total recall of the uniforms. Eventually, 164 attendants joined the suit.

By April 2013, more than 650 attendants, or 26 percent of the workforce at the time, had documented symptoms that their doctor thought were uniform related. In July, Alaska Airlines finally agreed to procure new interim uniforms from Lands' End but without admitting the uniforms had caused health issues. The new designs wouldn't arrive until March 2014, three years after attendants started getting sick. In the meantime, Alaska allowed airline attendants to buy and wear alternate uniforms but only if they could provide a doctor's note. John was released back to work by his workers' compensation doctor, with a restriction that he couldn't come in contact with the uniforms, a restriction that was impossible to meet—the majority of attendants were still wearing them.

When the new uniforms by Lands' End came in, the reports of reactions plummeted, and Anderson allowed herself to feel some measure of relief and accomplishment.

But John was permanently scarred, physically and emotionally. The former karate black belt walked slowly, nursing aching joint pain. Every day he wrapped his lesion-pocked arms in bandages. He was broke. Marco gave up his life in San Francisco to move to Long Beach to take care of him and to save his house from foreclosure.

Despite all this, John didn't let it control his life. Pictures from that time show him still smiling and laughing, and wearing funny hats, with his coworkers on holidays and birthdays. His hair had turned gray, and his damaged hands were covered in fingerless gloves so passengers wouldn't recoil as he handed them their soft drinks.

Mary developed multiple chemical sensitivity. She would get a migraine if she smelled paint fumes, cleaning products, exhaust fumes, or especially the de-icing fluid used on aircraft. When she walked onto a plane and felt her eyes starting to burn, she would know a fellow attendant had stored an old Twin Hill winter coat in the closet. Her eyes would be swollen for weeks afterward.

On October 3, 2016, Twin Hill announced that the judge had thrown out the Alaska attendants' case. "We were able to demonstrate to the Court, through rigorous testing supported by expert testimony, that our uniforms are safe and could not have caused the injuries these attendants claimed," the press release crowed. The court ruling cited the NIOSH report.

The attendants never got the chance to testify.

"It was gone so fast we didn't know what to do," Mary told me later. Once the judge refused to certify the lawsuit as a class action, Twin Hill offered the attendants in individual cases paltry settlements, threatening them with an astronomically-expensive legal fight if they didn't take the money and drop their cases. Only six stayed the course. (Twin Hill did not respond to my requests for comment.)

A judge ruled in Twin Hill's favor and ordered the six attendants to pay Twin Hill's attorneys' fees, which Mary says were in the hundreds of thousands of dollars. A new lawyer managed to get them out of the judgment, and they filed a suit against their former lawyer alleging malpractice, because, they claimed, he didn't adequately prepare the case or source expert testimony. A court date was scheduled for the malpractice suit, and then the pandemic caused the court to cancel it. A judge ruled against the attendants, again, without them ever getting their day in court.

Their fight for justice had come to an end.

It took a man to make American Airlines' leadership listen. In May 2017, in a town hall meeting between employees and leadership, AA pilot Joe Catan told the airline's president, Robert Isom, that his pilot's uniform was also giving him breathing problems, headaches, and rashes. "I do not have a safe environment in the cockpit," he said. Put on the spot by a respected male employee known for his competency under pressure (instead of legions of female and gay flight attendants who could be dismissed as hysterical drama queens), Isom hinted that the airline might give way.

The next month, American Airlines announced it would replace the uniforms.

The world's largest airline owned up in less than a year to what a massive failure the uniform rollout had been.

It's not like there were no red flags. According to Stewart Weltman, an attorney representing the American Airlines attendants, when American Airlines had conducted a wear test for its new Twin Hill uniforms with attendants in early 2016, attendants reported symptoms similar to the Alaska Airlines attendants.

"They forged ahead," Weltman told me. (American Airlines did not respond to my requests for comment.) A trickle of complaints to American Airlines headquarters that had started as soon as the boxes arrived at the homes of attendants and pilots turned into a flood within days of the official uniform rollout in September.

The Association of Flight Attendants doesn't represent

American Airlines attendants—as employees of the largest airline in the world, they have their own union: the Association of Professional Flight Attendants (APFA), which wouldn't talk to me because of ongoing litigation. But AFA industrial hygienist Judith Anderson was still in contact with US Airways attendants who had been absorbed into American Airlines when they finished merging the year before. AFA also represents attendants from three regional airlines that are owned by American and would have to wear the same uniforms: PSA, Piedmont, and Envoy.

So Anderson requested tests of fourteen pieces of the American Airlines flight attendant uniforms, which showed chromium, nickel, formaldehyde, the endocrine disruptors NPEO and OPEO, and suspected carcinogenic biocides pentachlorophenol, tetrachlorophenol, and trichlorophenol. They also contained chlordane, a pesticide so toxic that it was one of the very, very few substances that the EPA had banned for all uses in the United States in the late 1980s.

By May, one out of five American Airlines attendants had reported reactions, and the airline complained that though it had spent over $1 million trying to figure out which chemical in the Twin Hill uniforms was the problem, there was no one toxic chemical that could be fingered as the guilty party. Antimony, arsenic, cobalt, Disperse Red 60, Disperse Orange 30, and a variety of synthetic restricted substances with names only a chemist could hope to decipher—benzophenone, benzyl benzoate, 4-biphenyl ester benzoic acid, and 9,10-Dimethylanthracene—all were in at least one of the uniform pieces tested, and a few were over EU and Oeko-Tex limits, but no one chemical could be held responsible for the sheer variety and severity of reactions.

When American Airlines finally gave in, the fight wasn't quite over. Unfortunately, it would take until 2020 to give new, safer, Oeko-Tex-certified uniforms to the attendees. In the fall of 2017, forty attendants initiated a lawsuit against Twin Hill. As of October 2022, the case was still ongoing.

In January 2018, three years after it collected its survey data, Harvard finally published the results of its study of Alaska Airlines attendants. It found that after the introduction of the uniforms, the number of attendants with multiple chemical sensitivity, sore throats, cough, shortness of breath, itchy skin, rashes and hives, itchy eyes, loss of voice, and blurred vision had all more or less doubled. The study was unequivocal. "This study found a relationship between health complaints and the introduction of new uniforms."

One of the authors of the report, Dr. Irina Mordukhovich, had come to many of the same conclusions as Judith Anderson. "Each chemical that has been tested has been found to be below levels that would be considered an issue safety-wise," she told me later that year. "That being said, those levels themselves have been controversial. There's not necessarily a lot of evidence that goes into deciding what is a safe limit of a chemical. Even if each chemical is below thresholds that would be considered a direct safety issue, what we don't know is if you have hundreds of chemicals interacting together, what effects does that have?"

Unfortunately, the study had come two years too late for the Alaska attendants and linked the uniforms only to more immediate symptoms. It didn't have data on more serious, long-term illnesses like cancer and thyroid disease. And it didn't provide enough proof to force airlines like American, Delta, or Southwest to recall the uniforms, because it didn't show that just being around them—if you were a flight attendant who was allowed to wear a look-alike uniform—would also cause a debilitating reaction.

Even with the Harvard study, airlines and fashion brands still felt entitled to gaslight the thousands of attendants and pilots whose bodies were crying out for recognition of their pain.

"Flight attendants are the canary in the coal mine because of the length and consistency of their exposure," said Mordukhovich.

"They're working in these closed conditions with recirculated air, very low humidity; there are other potential contaminants in the aircraft; they have circadian rhythm disruption; there are a lot of factors that are simultaneously happening. That doesn't mean that other people in the population are not still being affected in some way. Let's say someone has clothing with the same components, they may not even notice; they just don't wear it so much."

In January 2020, Alaska Airlines announced it was rolling out Oeko-Tex-certified uniforms. John barely got to try his on. When the pandemic happened, all the airlines went into crisis mode, grounding planes and laying off workers. Judith Anderson was swept up in the drama of payroll cuts, plus keeping attendants safe from both COVID-19 and angry passengers who didn't want to wear a mask. With a deadly pandemic sweeping the globe, any momentum Anderson, the union, and the attendants had had in drawing attention to their plight of the toxic uniforms all but evaporated.

When, in May 2020, the Association of Flight Attendants released the results of tests it had done on Delta uniform pieces showing that three pieces all contained chromium—the red coat contained ten times the limit H&M allows on its own clothing— hardly anyone noticed.

John called Anderson to tell her he was taking the early retirement package that Alaska was offering its attendants. It was the end of a thirty-five-year career. He was in tears. "Thanks for being there," he told Anderson. "I'll keep pestering you. I'll keep in touch."

That was the last time she would speak to him. On February 22, 2021, John was climbing into bed beside Marco and grabbed his arm and said, "I can't breathe." Marco gave him his inhaler, and then his nebulizer, a small machine that turns medication into a breathable mist. He held it to John's mouth, but John slumped over. Marco hoped it was a joke. "That's not funny!" he shouted, slapping John, who came to and sucked in air from the nebulizer.

Marco was on the phone with 911 and jabbed John with an EpiPen. But by the time the paramedics arrived, he had stopped breathing. Twenty-five minutes of CPR failed to revive him. The official cause of death was cardiopulmonary arrest, secondary asthma. He was sixty-six years old.

I never got to talk to John myself. I had his name in a list of attendants who had sued their former lawyer for malpractice, but my search for such a common name pulled up nothing. Then, in the summer of 2021, I found his Facebook memorial page, and Marco's goodbye post. I messaged Marco, who agreed to get on the phone with me and talk about the lost love of his life. I spoke to him several times, for hours, oftentimes about his life as a single older man. He sounded sad and lonely, and angry.

He was mad at Twin Hill for making the uniforms. Mad at Alaska Airlines for gaslighting John. Mad at the company managing Alaska's employee benefits, which denied John care at every turn. Mad at the doctors who either dismissed John's symptoms or couldn't find a reason—or a solution—for his illness. Mad at the attendants who planned a big wake for John, and then disappeared, leaving Marco alone in his grief. Despite living an outwardly glamorous life, with friends inviting him on trips to Jordan and Mexico, Marco nursed the bitter flavor of losing a loved one for a senseless reason that no one had ever heard of, much less could understand.

"Nobody is even aware," Marco told me. "If you talk to a new flight attendant that joined Alaska in the last six, seven years, they say, *Oh, yeah, I heard about that. But that was a long time ago.* So it's all hush-hush and swept under the carpet. Whether the people that are really heavily affected are still around, or they have quit or have given up, I don't know."

———

Mary still works for Alaska Airlines. (She asked me to change identifying details so she wouldn't be fired.) "I fly a handful of days a month and that is it," she told me. She could get better if she removed herself completely from her triggers. But she can't quit—she needs the money. "With the illness, I have no energy. If I work one day, I have to count on not doing anything the next day. One day of work costs me one day to heal. I am depleting all of my bank accounts. All of my savings are being whittled away."

In 2021 alone, she mysteriously put on forty pounds. When I talked to her that October, she had a doctor's appointment to figure out why. Her thyroid levels were normal, though she said her inflammation markers were high.

I called her again in the summer of 2022 and filled her in on how the book was shaping up. I ran through the chapters, and when I mentioned autoimmune disease, she pounced. "Oh! Guess what happened since the last time we talked? I've been diagnosed with autoimmune diseases. Several."

After months of being given the runaround by white male doctors, she found a new one, a Black woman, who looked at her chart and immediately recognized the patterns. After some tests, Mary was diagnosed with mixed connective tissue disease, lupus, and Sjögren's.

It was still just anecdotal evidence, but how depressingly predictable. I wondered how many flight attendants are suffering in silence, unable to convince those around them that their symptoms are real, and that it was the uniforms that started all this. And how many more are on their way to an autoimmune disease diagnosis. This story won't be over for a very long time.

————

Tonya Osborne joined a case filed against Cintas in August 2020 as a lead plaintiff. The Southwest attendants seemed to have the best law firm in their corner: Girardi & Keese. Tom Girardi had been made famous by the Erin Brockovich movie and had a long history of winning huge class action "toxic torts" settlements for damage from exposure to chemicals and pollutants. If anyone could make Cintas pay for the ruinous effect the cheap uniforms had had on attendants' lives, it would be this firm.

Never mind. It came out in late 2020 that Girardi had misappropriated at least $2 million in client funds that were due to the families of those killed in the crash of a Boeing jet in Indonesia, much of it used to pay for the extensive wardrobe of his young wife, *Real Housewives of Beverly Hills* star Erika Jayne. Girardi was disbarred, the firm was thrown into chaos, and the other, smaller firms handling the case had to take over. The case was filed again in Ohio, where Cintas is based, in March 2021 and is awaiting class certification. Tonya's name is spelled wrong in the suit.

In the summer of 2022, Heather Poole from American Airlines noticed an uptick in activity in the Facebook group she created for attendants whose uniforms made them sick. It had been fairly quiet since American Airlines and Delta had both switched out their uniforms. Now, Southwest Airlines attendants flowed in. Mostly, they posted asking for advice on alternative uniforms. As several women told it, Southwest Airlines had created an Accommodations team to help attendants, but the approved look-alike dresses from brands like Lands' End, Old Navy, and Macy's were all sold out or not available in the correct size. As of October 2022, Southwest had not yet announced that it would replace the uniforms, and it did not respond to my questions.

I caught up with Tonya in October 2022. She had just gotten out of the hospital from another surgery and then a bowel obstruction the week before, and had been told by the doctors that she also had lupus and Crohn's, along with the three other autoimmune diseases she was already dealing with. She was surviving on social security payments of $1,300 a month.

"Alden, I'm so tired and I have to get a job but my body hurts," she texted me. I expressed my condolences.

"PBA . . . prolly be alright," she texted back.

On December 24, 2021, I flashed my vaccination card to a Delta employee manning the self-check-in terminals at JFK. When I made it to the gate, I was surprised to see two women clicking down the terminal in bright red coats and purple pants. As I boarded the plane, I asked a male attendant, who was dressed in gray and handing out sanitizer wipes, if the new uniforms had been distributed yet. He looked at me in surprise, no doubt wondering how I knew. "The nonpurple ones," I elucidated.

"No, they haven't arrived. Only some pieces, the skirt, I think."

"Supply-chain issues?"

"Yeah. Covid and whatnot." He shrugged.

Later, another silver-haired male attendant dressed in a black suit offered me pretzels. I asked him if he had had a reaction to the uniforms. He told me, leaning close and talking over the pilot announcement, that the uniform had given him a terrible rash and nosebleeds. Did he have a reaction to his colleagues' uniforms? Yes—he lifted a hand to his temple—brain fog and migraines.

I texted Chingy Wong and another, older Delta attendant who I'll call Helen, who was run out of her position when she refused to wear the toxic uniforms any longer. I thought they both must be so frustrated, thinking there was light at the end of the tunnel and yet waiting in plum-colored purgatory. They both responded. Apparently, some attendants had posted on Facebook that the new, Oeko-Tex-approved uniforms were also causing reactions.

In September, the Association of Flight Attendants, which had been trying to unionize Delta attendants, released the results of the tests it had commissioned on the new, Oeko-Tex-certified uniforms. While these new uniforms were much better than the Passport Plum ones, a pair of men's "untreated" non-wool pants had tetrachloroethylene (PCE for short) slightly above the Oeko-Tex limit. Two ladies' scarves that were tested had between two and seven times the recommended limit for chromium. Some of the suit pants and skirts contained tetrachloroethylene (TCE), styrene, and toluene—"all at levels below or barely above the fabric limits."

For a "normal" person, these uniforms would probably be okay to wear. But it makes sense, given what I had learned throughout reporting the book, that a person who has TILT—who has been overexposed and now reacts to a tiny amount of certain common fashion chemicals—would not be able to wear them without having a reaction.

Delta Air Lines emailed me this statement in October of 2022: "At Delta, the safety and wellbeing of our employees and customers is, and will always be, our number one priority. We are proud to offer our flight attendants a complete collection of untreated, STANDARD 100 by OEKO-TEX® uniform pieces, which means that the pieces have been certified free of harmful substances. At the same time, we are continuing to engage in the accommodation process to provide alternative options for flight attendants with verified medical restrictions."

In the summer of 2022, Helen texted me to say she had developed skin cancer on her nipple. Chingy, a month later, emailed me to say Delta had finally fired her, citing too many unexcused absences.

I was confused as to why Chingy was upset, because she had every reason to say *good riddance*. A combination of psychotherapy, treatment by a functional doctor, and avoiding the chemicals that have been shown to make her sick meant her symptoms were under control. She had been splitting her time between working in a hospital and attending school to become a nurse. She was even engaged to be married! Everything seemed to be going well for her. Why would she even want her job back?

"I want to be compensated for what they did to me," she said. "Every time I have a reaction, it reminds me of Delta. It makes me so angry. I was healthy and now I'm not. It's a part of me. I'm working with my therapist but it's so hard to let go and forgive.

"I'm reminiscing about the good parts of the job, and I can't let it go."

───

While she was collecting unemployment during the pandemic, Jaclyn took some classes on fashion sustainability at the Fashion Institute of Technology (FIT). "I was having a very hard personal time. I was just like, *What is my purpose? Will I ever find a job again?* It was a really dark point in my life. I couldn't find a job and my hair was falling out. I didn't feel confident." A yoga teacher told her, "Maybe you shouldn't be looking for the same production job. What is it about fashion that you love? What brings you joy?"

The answer was vintage fashion. Jaclyn got her flea market vendor license and started selling at the Brooklyn Flea. Her hair started to grow back. When I spoke to her in October 2022, she had just gotten her first haircut in years. "My health is great," she said. "I'm fully in remission."

I realized that I hadn't shared with her all the things I had learned since I first spoke to her nearly a year before. So I explained what the Duke research had found about disperse dyes, one of the several fashion substances the patch test had confirmed she's allergic to, and how even people who don't work in fashion are ingesting and breathing them in from house dust. I explained how mast cells work, and Claudia Miller's theory that once triggered, they're the biological mechanism behind chemical intolerance. I told her how—though genetics are important when it comes to who is predisposed to developing certain illnesses—research points to autoimmune diseases being largely tied to environmental causes, including chemicals.

She interrupted me before I could even finish. "I worked in the fashion industry for eighteen years," she reminded me. Along with her digestive issues, she had severe scalp psoriasis, another type of autoimmune skin condition. She told me the smell of strong perfume can make her vomit. The signs were there, if she had known what to look for.

"I think what you're saying, it all makes sense. I think it's all connected. Two and a half years ago I was falling apart. Like with any autoimmune disease, it's like you don't even know why these things are happening or what's causing it. And that's so frustrating, trying to figure out what is actually going on and pinpoint it and then figure out what treatment will work, which takes so long. And, you know, it's like, me not being around chemicals and working in production and having that stress, and touching the clothes all day and every day . . . I'm not having the symptoms anymore."

"That's the biggest lesson I learned from all of this—to tune in when your body's sending these wake-the-fuck-up calls," she had told me many months earlier. "Like, the skin reactions, I got the test. And then I did nothing, and I kept it moving. And then, you know, I felt like someone was stabbing me with knives. It took me four days, until I could barely walk, to go and do anything. Same thing with the Crohn's; I saw the signs, and I ignored them for months until it was like, *Your organs are failing, you're gonna die.* In the pandemic, being put on furlough and having that extra time and all of my hair falling out and not even wanting to go into the world, because I didn't even recognize who I was? I really started to take a step back and be like, *Is this making me happy?*

"It's just scary . . . to have a set salary for so many years to take the step to do what you love," she said. "It's so risky, without having the financial security or a partner, or someone that I can fall back on. But I've never been happier. I feel like I'm finally doing what I love."

I should say that this is a moving anecdote, but it's not evidence. I went in search of a researcher who could confirm my thoroughly unscientific hunch based on all the bleeding-edge research I had excavated, and only got a bracing dose of *maybe*.

"I think that you just should be aware that it's not a conventional view. Maybe that's why you're writing a book about it," said Dr. Marc E. Rothenberg, director of the Division of Allergy and Immunology and the Bunning Professor of Pediatrics at Cincinnati Children's Hospital, when I got him on the phone to ask. "It would be very highly disregarded in the medical community, but probably very welcomed by the lay community to think that there's environmental things like chemicals that are causing these things.

"Most people would say that there's not direct proof on that, but it is a theory that probably needs more research."

So yes, I could be proven completely wrong by the further research that we so badly need. If so, I'll accept that in exchange for some clarity—and more good ideas on how we can solve these overlapping problems.

In October 2022, I checked in with Debbie from Gloversville via email, asking about her family's health. Last we spoke, her little brother had just had what doctors thought was a heart attack, and her mother had early-stage colon cancer and had cysts in her breasts removed. I hoped Debbie had good news to share.

"Here are my updates," she wrote back in her remarkably matter-of-fact way. "Since we spoke last, my older brother passed away from a heart attack. I didn't mention him during our interview because we didn't know he had a heart condition. My little brother (the one I mentioned in the interview) has been in and out of the hospital for testing, but has stayed pretty stable. He definitely has a heart condition . . . just working on trying to get his health back. My older sister (I believe I mentioned her in our interview) [has] been in and out of the hospital the past 6 months with at least 2 strokes. She has had a few visits with her oncologist and is still cancer free. I found out that my father has testicular cancer. He told my [older] sister. He and I have not been on speaking terms for years so I haven't confirmed that; but I'm sure it's true based on his actions of trying to reconnect with all of his children. My mother's health hasn't changed."

Debbie went on to write that she has polyps again, but they're not cancerous. They're being monitored.

"I have to say that I think of you and our conversation every time I eat something that tastes off/chemically or when I smell the chemicals on clothes. I know others think I'm nuts. All I can do is laugh it off. My eating habits have definitely changed. . . . more fresh foods; and less processed and less meat. I had a potted garden on my back deck this year; and bought a lot from local farmers. I canned as much as I could so I have it once winter hits and I can't get the same quality in the stores."

I was very affected by this email, which is a whole roller-coaster ride of emotions, wrapped neatly up in packaging of equanimity and frankness. She had lost another family member and had multiple health scares with other family members, all in the previous year. And yet, she had found some measure of faith and control over her own life with a few lifestyle tweaks that sounded so wholesome. It couldn't hurt, right? To grow a little garden and do some canning? I found myself being happy for her, despite it all. At the very least, I was definitely rooting for her. I wrote back and said I wanted to come meet her someday soon.

———

I have no doubt that I will hear more stories of clothing chemistry gone wrong. In fact, before this book was even finished, the copy editor wrote an alarming story right in the margins. Her father-in-law, ever vigilant about sun exposure and skin cancer, had bought an Australian leather "bush" hat in 2019 off the Internet to wear during his walks and bike rides in his home country of France—he wore it once or twice a week for a couple of hours. Though it came from Australia, he didn't know where it was made or where the leather was tanned.

"The Australian hat soon started to puzzle me," he wrote to me by email, with help translating from his wife and his daughter-in-law, the copy editor. "Each time I wore it, I noticed that it left a reddish band on my forehead. One day in 2021, I observed that a pimple located on the red band produced by the hat would not heal despite my frequently dabbing it with alcohol. I decided I needed to check with my dermatologist, who treated it with nitrogen. That didn't do a thing to it. Sometime later, I went back to her office, and she concluded after examination that it was cancer!"

His doctor prescribed him two creams for treatment, and he seemed healed until February 2022, when another small pimple turned out to be cancerous and treatment started again. Six months later, he was still anxious. "I have been very stressed and worried about the possibility of the cancer spreading. The dermatologist and I think that these tumors were caused by the chemicals used in the tanning of the leather of the hat.

"I hope my story may alert others to the dangers of chemicals on clothing and gear."

———

The story of clothing chemicals doesn't end in our closets. Oh, no. The "end" is often far away, in a sandy pile on a beach in Africa, a desert in Chile, a leaky landfill in Malaysia, or in your tap water.

I put "end" in quotes, because really, we don't know when or if the end will come for these chemicals and plastic materials.

PFAS, as I said before, is what scientists call "persistent." It doesn't break down, instead circulating around and around our globe, forever. I've had several EcoCult readers email me asking how they can responsibly dispose of their old outdoor gear, with its durable water repellent. My answer is, unfortunately, you can't. PFAS will leach out in landfills and contaminate anything that is made from these recycled fabrics. Traditional incineration of clothing that has PFAS doesn't make it go away; it just spreads these perfluorinated chemicals through the air to surrounding communities.

In August 2022, however, some good news broke. Scientists have found a way to break down PFAS just by adding some sodium hydroxide—otherwise known as lye. Combined with some proven techniques for filtering PFAS out of water, the news provided some much-needed hope for cleaning it out of our environment. The only thing is, we can't douse our homes or all our clothing with lye. So we can't let brands use this as an excuse to keep slathering it all over our belongings.

Fortunately, as a society, we seem to be moving toward a future without PFAS. In August 2022, the EPA proposed designating certain PFAS chemicals as hazardous substances, for the purpose of monitoring their emissions and holding manufacturers accountable for cleaning them up out of our environment. ZDHC announced in September that it was adding all PFAS to its manufacturing restricted substance list, meaning member brands and suppliers will have to get it out of their formulations and textiles by November 2023. And in October, California governor Gavin Newsom signed into law a ban on PFAS in makeup, personal care products, and textiles. It will go into effect in 2025 for most fabrics, but outdoor apparel brands will have until 2028 to get PFAS out of their textiles.

Plastic is also going to be around for a while. Scientists have hazarded a guess that plastic materials such as polyester and nylon will take around four hundred years to degrade completely. And if it's in our environment, it's in us. Microplastics and microfibers have been found in placentas, in human blood, in our lungs. We must do much more research on the link between microfibers and our health, but a 2022 study found that people who have inflammatory bowel disease tend to have more microplastics present in their feces.

We also are doing a terrible job of responsibly disposing of our old clothing. In Cambodia, according to a 2022 investigation, factories ship the waste from garment factories to brick kilns, where they burn it for fuel. A kiln worker told *Unearthed* that he suffers from nosebleeds, and his father died at age fifty-one. Labels from

Nike, Reebok, Michael Kors, Diesel, and Ralph Lauren were found in the piles.

In conscious fashion campaigner Maxine Bédat's 2021 book *Unraveled: The Life and Death of a Garment*, she finds herself in a burning Ghanaian landfill, with plumes of toxic smoke billowing around her, filled with whatever had been in the old Nikes, H&M clothing, and fake Versace bags piled in the muck.

How did that clothing make it to Ghana? Well, according to Bédat's research, 4.8 percent of all the trash Americans threw away in 2017 was clothes and shoes, almost 12.8 million tons of it. If you're muttering to yourself that you don't throw clothing away, you *donate* it, I'm sorry, but many of those donations are also ending up in the trash and environment for reasons outside your control. For more than a decade, the estimate has been that 80 percent of what we donate is shipped overseas because Americans are simply uninterested in out-of-date clothing—it's easier to buy new fast fashion for the same price as, or even cheaper than, old stuff.

But data from the Salvation Army is even bleaker: in its largest New York store, only 8 percent of the garments that are donated are sold in store. "Every year the United States exports more than a billion pounds of used clothing," Bédat wrote. "Data from 2016 shows that of all the world's secondhand clothing, 40 percent comes from just three countries: the United States (15 percent), the United Kingdom (13 percent), and Germany (11 percent). Together the EU and US represent 65 percent of the value of global used clothing exports." And China, with its growing middle and upper classes, is catching up.

Much of that old clothing is shipped to Ghana. An estimated fifteen million items flow through the huge Kantamanto Market in Accra each week, and the quality of what we ship over has been dropping like a stone. It's becoming cheaper, and more prone to be stained, moldy, and ripped garbage that no one would pay even twenty-five cents for. An estimated seventy-seven tons of unsold clothing is collected by the Accra Metropolitan Assembly six days per week and deposited in the city's main landfill. But that represents only about 25 percent of Kantamanto's total waste. "Another 15 percent is picked up by private, informal collectors who may illegally dump it in waterways, bury it on beaches, burn it in open lots, or simply leave it along the side of the road," Bédat explains.

Whether Ghanaians are getting cancer or autoimmune disease from breathing in smoky air and drinking water contaminated by the chemicals in old clothing, we may never know. Like the low-income communities in the United States who live close to defunct dye factories and reside in lead-contaminated homes, there are too many variables for us to ever prove that link.

This vast web of invisible chemicals that stretches from a chemical factory in India, to a dyehouse in China, to a store in New Jersey, and then back over the ocean to a market in Ghana is what some now call a *hyperobject*. When I read this new term close to the end of my year of research and travel across the globe, trying to connect the tiny hidden dots, I felt it in my soul. A hyperobject is a new term for a thing we can never see in its entirety. It is too pervasive and huge for you to influence; it's something that seems—like climate change or the global economy—to be incomprehensible while also controlling our lives, often in a menacing sense.

But I don't want you to lose hope. Because you *can* start to take control—today, right now. It requires only that you value yourself and your health above TikTok trends and "easy-care" marketing promises. Take a deep breath before you buy. See if you can find it secondhand, from your community. Value traditional, natural fibers. Spread the word.

Maybe, just maybe, we can start to make a change.

GLOSSARY

1,2-Dichloroethane—Also known as ethylene dichloride; used as a solvent and to produce vinyl chloride and PVC. A 2017 Swedish study found ethylene dichloride fumes at thirty times the occupational exposure limits in a container of shoes. (p. 183)

4-Phenylenediamine (PPD)—Aromatic amine used in the production of azo dye and known skin allergen. Often found in black rubber products and black hair and fur dye. Acute exposure to high levels may cause severe dermatitis, eye irritation, asthma, gastritis, renal failure, vertigo, tremors, convulsions, and coma. Long-term exposure can cause eczema-like skin rashes. (p. 38)

Acrylic—Synthetic textile fiber often used to simulate wool fiber in knitwear. (pp. 36, 76, 215)

AFIRM—The Apparel and Footwear International RSL Management Group. A membership organization of apparel and footwear companies that collaborate to create a restricted substance list (RSL) and provide guidance to fashion brands on risk management and testing for hazardous chemicals in consumer fashion products. (pp. 213–14)

Alkylphenol ethoxylates (APEOs)—Can be used as or found in dozens of different fashion manufacturing substances and processes, including detergents, spinning oils, softeners, emulsifying/dispersing agents for dyes and prints, degumming for silk production, dyes and pigment preparations, plus polyester and down fillings. APEOs are often found on wool fashion products but as of 2021 are prohibited from use throughout Europe's fashion supply chain, due to EU regulation. (pp. 119, 123, 225)

Amines—A class of basic organic (carbon-containing) chemical compounds that are used in the production of chemical substances like synthetic azo dyes, and can be released from azo dyes when they come into contact with our skin. Exposure to certain arylamines, especially among factory workers, has been linked to cancer. (pp. 42, 53, 81, 100, 166, 192, 225)

Analytical standards—A chemical compound of high purity and known concentration used in lab tests as a reference. (pp. 44, 222, 223)

Aniline dyes—The first synthetic dyes invented, made from amines synthesized from coal tar. Have since been phased out of fashion. (pp. 100–102, 105–106, 109, 110–12, 122)

Antimony—A metalloid often used in fashion as a flame retardant or as a catalyst in polyester production. Has been found in children's clothing and airline uniforms. (pp. 26, 63, 123, 203, 235)

Arsenic—A highly toxic, naturally occuring chemical element. Has been phased out of use in dyes, but sometimes is found as a contaminant in fashion products. (pp. 26, 55, 63, 66, 95, 96, 97–99, 101, 106, 119, 120, 123, 147, 192, 202, 225, 235)

Autoimmune disease—When the body's immune system can't tell the difference between harmful invading cells and the body's own cells, leading the immune system to attack one's own body. There are more than eighty autoimmune diseases; psoriasis, multiple sclerosis, Hashimoto's thyroiditis, and fibromyalgia are commonly known ones. Researchers believe that autoimmune diseases are likely caused by a combination of genetic predisposition and environmental triggers like toxins and viruses. (pp. 1, 5, 9, 35, 43, 69, 125, 148–52, 154–55, 229, 239, 240, 243–44, 250)

Azo dyes—A large class of synthetic dyes. Twenty-two azo dyes are banned in the European Union because they have been shown to release carcinogenic and mutagenic amines when in contact with our skin bacteria. (pp. 6, 37, 38, 40, 42–43, 44, 45, 51, 52, 53, 104, 112, 148, 170, 171, 174, 175, 177, 189, 192, 196, 204, 207, 224)

Benzene—A carcinogenic chemical used as a solvent in dyehouses and in adhesive production. (pp. 84, 100, 101, 138, 183, 192, 218, 224)

Benzidine—A carcinogenic chemical connected to bladder cancer in dye factory workers. Because they cleave into carcinogenic amines, benzidine-based azo dyes have been banned in multiple countries and are no longer produced or used commercially in the US, though they have still shown up in fashion products. (pp. 103, 111, 185)

Benzophenone—Mutagen, carcinogen, and endocrine disruptor. Despite being banned for use in food products and packaging in the United States, and in personal care products in California, benzophenone was found in a 2022 study in the urine of American women, and ranks in the top twenty chemicals for production volume. While rare in fashion, it has also been found in airline uniforms and in 2012 tests by Greenpeace of everyday apparel. (pp. 122, 235)

Beta-naphthylamine (BNA)—Ingredient in dye production. Linked to bladder cancer in dye factory workers. (p. 111)

Bisphenol A—A chemical used in the production of plastics and potent endocrine disruptor. Some products containing BPA have been banned or voluntarily phased out in the European Union and several other developed countries. In some cases, it has been replaced with other chemicals in the same class, such as BPS and BPF, which research shows have similar health effects. (pp. 119, 122, 124, 224, 225, 227)

Bluesign—A Swiss company that provides advisory services to brands and retailers, chemical suppliers, and manufacturers. The bluesign label verifies that a product or facility has been audited and found to be up to bluesign's standards of chemical safety. (pp. 196, 207, 214)

Brominated flame retardants—Chemical flame retardants containing the element bromine. Heavily regulated and phased out of use on fashion products. (pp. 40, 91, 148)

Carcinogenic—Has the potential to cause cancer. (pp. 5, 10, 26, 42, 76, 81, 92, 94, 100, 112, 120, 166, 174, 183, 192, 193, 199, 218, 225, 228, 235)

CAS Registry Number—Because many chemicals have multiple names, the US-based Chemical Abstracts Service assigns a unique number to every publicly listed chemical substance, for easy identification. When it comes to chemical products and their ingredient lists, these identification numbers are not normally shared with factories, fashion brands, or consumers, as chemical companies deem them proprietary information.

Chemical—While many laypeople use the word *chemical* to denote a synthetic substance that has hazardous properties, a chemical is any substance that has a defined composition, from H_2O and CO_2 to man-made chemicals like phthalates and perfluorooctanoic acid (PFOA).

Chemical classes—Chemicals that have similar structures, indicating they might act similarly when it comes to human toxicity. Examples include bisphenols (BPA, BPS) and PFAS (per- and polyfluoroalkyl substances such as PFOA and PFOS). Some researchers and advocates hope to have chemicals regulated as classes to prevent regrettable substitution. (p. 52)

Chlorinated paraffins, short-chain—Persistent, bioaccumulative, and toxic to aquatic organisms at low concentrations. Have been found in animals, as well as samples of human breast milk from Canada, Europe, and Japan. May be used as softeners or flame retardants in leather production, or as a plasticizer in plastic and faux leather and rubber production. Restricted for use in fashion but found in fashion products imported to the EU such as flip-flops. (p. 192)

Cobalt—Natural element that is part of vitamin B_{12}, which is required for animal and human health at low amounts. Excessive and chronic exposure can cause neurological and endocrine health issues. Used in dyes and pigments to create blue. (pp. 26, 235)

Consumer Product Safety Commission (CPSC)—An independent agency of the United States federal government that promotes the safety of consumer products through safety standards, testing, research, and product recalls. (pp. 9, 24, 41, 55, 78, 174, 182, 183, 184, 185, 186, 188, 223–24)

Cradle to Cradle (C2C)—An institute and certification promoting circularity, safety, and sustainability in consumer products. (pp. 196, 228)

Crohn's disease—A type of serious inflammatory bowel disease. While Crohn's was formerly attributed to stress and diet, many researchers and physicians believe it is an autoinflammatory disease that presents after an intestinal infection allows allergens into the lining of the bowel, making the gut intolerant to those and similar substances. (pp. 48, 50, 151)

Cytokines—Tiny proteins secreted by mast cells that provide signaling to the immune system. (pp. 136, 137)

Dermatitis—A general term for skin irritation, including everything from dry and itchy skin to rashes, flaking, and oozing. Contact dermatitis is caused by something touching the skin and is a common diagnosis for those with textile allergies. (pp. 24, 28, 46, 110, 125)

Dimethylacetamide (DMAc)—Solvent used in elastane. High and repeated exposure can cause neurological problems and liver damage. (p. 203)

Dimethylformamide (DMFa)—Solvent used in plastics, rubber, and polyurethane. Classified as reproductive toxic and can be toxic to the liver. Some brands restrict its use in fashion production.

Dimethyl fumarate (DMF)—Antifungal that is banned in the European Union for use in consumer products because it is a skin sensitizer and respiratory irritant. May contaminate clothing through sachets in packaging to prevent mold buildup during shipping. (p. 26)

Dimethylol dihydroxyethylene urea (DMDHEU)—Resin invented to attach substances that provide performance qualities to cotton. Can degrade and release formaldehyde. (p. 80)

DINCH (1,2-Cyclohexane dicarboxylic acid diisononyl ester)—A plasticizer promoted as a safer alternative to phthalates. Was found in the urine of American women in a 2022 study and has been linked in one study to lower fertility in women. (p. 122)

Disperse dyes—A class of dyes that penetrate synthetic fibers such as polyester, acetate, and polyamide. Many disperse dyes are restricted because they are allergens and are frequently included in patch tests for allergies. Azo disperse dyes were the subject of recent research out of Duke University that found high amounts in house dust and polyester children's clothing. (pp. 26, 31, 38, 40, 42, 43, 44–45, 51, 52, 53, 148, 153, 171, 177, 213, 217, 220, 243)

Drop-shipping—Notorious practice of shipping low-quality products straight from the factory (usually in Asia) to the customer, with no retailer in between. Is often made possible by social media ads. It can take up to two weeks for the package to arrive, and it generally doesn't go through the same

customs and border safety checks that typical fashion shipments go through, making it a tempting strategy for ultra-
fast-fashion brands without chemical management policies.
(p. 212)

Eczema—a.k.a. atopic dermatitis. A condition of dry, itchy, and
inflamed skin. Though it can occur at any age, it often shows
up on children's skin. (pp. 47, 52, 54, 104, 108, 110, 126, 140,
151, 162, 218)

Endocrine disruptor—Interferes with your hormones, which in
turn impact all the important systems in your body: immunological, metabolic, neurological, and cardiovascular. They
have more serious health consequences for children and pregnant women. Includes PFAS, BPA, and phthalates. (pp. 6, 22,
32, 78, 91, 120–21, 122, 123, 127, 152, 203, 225, 231, 235)

Environmental Protection Agency (EPA)—An independent executive agency of the United States federal government tasked
with regulating exposure to toxic substances in the air and
water. (pp. 4, 41, 78, 84, 85, 87, 89, 93, 112, 176, 189, 190,
199, 204, 216, 218, 219, 235, 248)

Ethyl acrylate—Sensitizer. Used to manufacture plastics and
paints for textile coatings. (p. 38)

Fluorine—A chemical element. At high amounts (100 ppm or
more) its presence on a textile likely indicates that PFAS were
intentionally added. (pp. 91–92, 198, 223)

Formaldehyde—A naturally occurring chemical compound that
at high exposure levels has been linked to cancer. Often found
in textiles and other fashion products, especially performance
textiles that are antiwrinkle. (pp. 18, 21, 29, 55, 72, 80, 81, 84,
85, 86, 120, 122, 132, 138, 140, 171, 183, 192, 193, 201, 203,
204, 225, 235)

Genotoxic—Chemical agents that damage the genetic material in
an organism, which may lead to cancer. All mutagens are
genotoxic, but some genotoxic substances are not mutagenic.
(p. 42)

GOTS—Global Organic Textile Standard. A certification and label that covers various aspects of textile production, including safe chemistry. (pp. 167, 196, 214)

Green chemistry—A practice of designing chemical products so that they have reduced or no hazardous substances from the outset.

Hazardous—When used to describe chemicals, anything that causes physical or health harm. (pp. 10, 44, 93, 166, 168, 169, 170, 172, 183, 197, 213, 214, 218, 221, 223, 224, 227, 248)

Heavy metal—Defined as a metal with a high density or high atomic weight. Many can cause toxicity—or heavy metal poisoning—including arsenic, lead, mercury, and chromium. (pp. 26, 63, 65, 66, 67, 123, 125, 139, 147, 152, 173, 174, 192, 201)

Hexavalent chromium—A carcinogenic heavy metal often used in leather tanning. Can also be used as a dyeing additive, and dye-fixing and color-fastness treatment, especially in wool products. (pp. 26, 75, 192)

Hohenstein—A well-respected German lab that tests fashion products and materials for hazardous and restricted substances. Can test to Oeko-Tex standards. (pp. 27, 196, 197, 198, 199, 200, 203, 204, 205, 206)

Industrial hygienist—A science professional or engineer who conducts safety and health investigations to prevent workplace exposures that would lead to illness or injury. (pp. 18, 20, 26, 67, 96, 235)

Interstitial lung disease—Called flock worker's lung when it breaks out in synthetic velvet factories. Caused by inhalation of hazardous dust. (pp. 151, 164)

Lead—A toxic heavy metal that is heavily regulated in many countries in consumer products, including in children's products in the United States. In fashion, it can be most often found in paints and coatings. Can cause serious and permanent neurological damage, especially in children. (pp. 26, 43, 46, 63, 119,

123, 125, 147, 162, 174, 184, 185, 186, 192, 193, 202, 212, 223, 225, 250)

Manufacturing restricted substance list (MRSL)—A list created by ZDHC of chemical substances that should not be used intentionally in facilities that produce for fashion brands and retailers. (pp. 166, 169, 214, 248)

Mass spectrometry—A scientific technique used in analytical chemistry to measure the mass-to-charge ratio of charged particles. The latest mass spectrometry technology and techniques can be used to identify all the chemical substances present in a sample and their chemical structure. This is a more holistic approach than traditional testing methods, which test for different chemicals one by one and require prior knowledge of what chemicals—out of thousands of possibilities—to look for. (pp. 41, 42, 44, 45, 201, 223)

Mast cell activation syndrome—When a person experiences repeated and often debilitating allergic reactions such as hives, brain fog, and fatigue. Caused by the mast cells releasing immunological-regulating chemicals too much and too often. In many cases, the name is used interchangeably with TILT and multiple chemical sensitivity. (pp. 9, 133, 137, 138, 143)

Mercury—Toxic heavy metal used for several hundred years to make hats. When it comes to fashion, today it's most often found in paints. Can cause serious neurological issues and tremors. (pp. 61, 63, 66–69, 119, 123, 147, 190, 194, 225)

Multiple chemical sensitivity—Similar to mast cell activation syndrome; when a person experiences reactions in several systems of the body—skin rashes and hives, brain fog, fatigue, breathing problems—in response to exposure to synthetic fragrances and other chemicals. (pp. 9, 133, 134, 233, 236)

Mutagenic—A chemical that can permanently change genetic material in an organism, potentially leading to birth defects. All mutagens are genotoxic, but some genotoxic substances are not mutagenic. (pp. 10, 42, 192, 228)

National Institute for Occupational Safety and Health (NIOSH)—An organization that researches work-related injury and illness and makes recommendations on how to prevent them. (pp. 25, 28, 233)

Nitrobenzene—A toxic chemical made from benzene as a precursor to aniline and benzidine. Formerly used in shoe blacking. (pp. 100, 102, 108, 110)

Nonylphenol ethoxylate (NPE)—A subset of APEOs; an endocrine disruptor often used to scour fat and oils off textiles. Prohibited for use in the supply chain as of 2021 but often found on wool products. (pp. 6, 123, 166)

Nylon—Generic description for synthetic polyamide textiles made from petroleum. Popular for outdoor and performance textiles, bathing suits, and carpeting. (pp. 7, 53, 76, 215, 248)

Occupational Safety and Health Administration (OSHA)—A large regulatory agency of the United States Department of Labor that sets and enforces workplace safety standards, including safe levels of chemical exposure. (pp. 19, 25, 77, 204)

Oeko-Tex—A nonprofit organization linked to the for-profit Hohenstein lab with a suite of labels certifying that a material has been tested in an accredited lab and deemed free of their list of hazardous substances. (pp. 27, 51, 120, 167, 170, 196, 197–99, 203, 204, 205, 206, 207, 214, 235, 237, 241, 242)

Organic chemistry—Not to be confused with the practice of growing crops without the use of pesticides; in the field of chemistry, denotes chemical substances containing carbon, which can be from plant, animal, or fossil sources. Organic chemicals range from perfectly safe to very toxic.

Organotins—A large class of chemicals that combine organic chemicals with tin substances. Look for substances that end in *-yltin*, such as tetraethyltin, dibutyltin, dioctyltin, monobutyltin, and so on. Some are known endocrine disruptors. Most often associated with biocides and pesticides, but in fashion can be found in plastics, rubber, inks, paints, metallic glitter, polyurethane products, and heat transfer prints. (pp. 123, 204)

Particle-induced gamma-ray emission (PIGE)—A type of nuclear analysis that can be used to identify the presence and amount of inorganic chemicals in consumer products, such as total fluorine at a level likely indicating the presence of intentionally added perfluorinated chemicals (PFAS) in a test pioneered by physicist Graham Peaslee at Notre Dame. (pp. 91, 223)

Patch test—A dermatologist-administered test that places up to eighty patches containing common allergens on a patient to ascertain which might be causing an allergic reaction. (pp. 38, 51, 55, 132, 141, 145, 218, 232, 243)

Per- and polyfluoroalkyl substances (PFAS)—A class of man-made chemicals invented in the mid-twentieth century that provides water repellency and stain resistance to a wide range of consumer products, including textiles. Includes long-chain PFOA and PFOS, along with thousands of other types of short-chain perfluorinated chemicals. The commonly known brand names are Gore-Tex and Teflon. (pp. 31, 85, 86, 88, 89, 91–93, 111, 119, 121, 122, 123, 125, 126, 166, 167, 171, 189, 191, 198–99, 204, 205–206, 213, 215, 220, 222, 224, 225, 226–27, 247–48)

PFOA, PFOS—Long-chain perfluorinated chemicals with eight or more carbon atoms. Have been definitively linked to cancer, are suspected endocrine disruptors, and are persistent and bioaccumulative. Some products containing these chemicals have been banned in the EU and voluntarily phased out in the United States. (pp. 86, 87, 88, 89, 224, 227)

Phthalates—Chemicals known as plasticizers that are used in plastics, including polyester and PVC. They are known endocrine disruptors and some are subject to regulation in the

European Union and United States. (pp. 5, 6, 54, 78, 119–20, 122, 123, 124, 125, 152, 166, 173, 174, 184, 192, 193, 202, 212, 223, 224, 225)

Plasticizers—Chemical substances added to a synthetic resin to make it softer and more flexible. The majority are phthalates that are added to PVC to make it flexible. (pp. 122)

Polycyclic aromatic hydrocarbons (PAHs)—A natural component of crude oil—which all end in *-ene*, from acenaphthene to pyrene—can be found in rubbers, plastics, lacquers, and coatings, especially in outsoles of footwear and screen prints. PAHs can be in carbon black or show up in recycled materials. They are carcinogenic, and animal studies link them to blood, immune system, reproductive, neurological, and developmental effects. (p. 122)

Polyester—A synthetic fiber that makes up half the textiles used in fashion today. Also known as polyethylene terephthalate, or PET, it's the same material used to make plastic water bottles. (pp. 7, 16, 26, 31, 38, 40, 41, 45, 48, 52, 53, 76, 80, 122, 123, 145, 153, 165, 170, 171, 184, 215, 217, 248)

Polyurethane (PU)—A synthetic material often used in fashion as a leather substitute. (pp. 53, 76, 89, 126, 171, 200, 215)

Polyvinyl chloride (PVC)—A plastic material that is often either clear or used as a cheap leather alternative. Notoriously toxic because of the off-gassing of vinyl chloride, which is linked to Raynaud's and scleroderma, plus a variety of cancers. Also often contains endocrine-disrupting phthalates to make it pliable and soft. (pp. 55, 72, 76, 77, 78, 120, 200, 215)

Potassium dichromate—A type of hexavalent chromium and commonly-used salt for leather tanning, dyeing, and waterproofing fabrics. Toxic and a very common allergen. (p. 101)

Prop 65—Legislation in California that requires brands to put a warning label on any product containing toxic chemicals like formaldehyde, lead, cadmium, some phthalates, and BPA. If someone discovers through testing that a product contains one of these substances, yet doesn't come with a label saying it's carcinogenic or reproductive toxic, they can file a notice with California and then sue. (pp. 92, 193–94)

Psoriasis—A chronic autoimmune condition of a rash with itchy, scaly patches. There is no cure, but it can be managed. (pp. 50, 148, 243)

PubChem—Open-source database of chemicals and their human toxicity that is managed by the US federal agency the National Institutes of Health. (p. 44)

Pulmonary sarcoidosis—Inflammation of the lungs. Researchers suspect the cause of this rare condition is related to inhaling chemicals. (p. 151)

Quinoline dyes—A type of disperse dye no longer in use. Quinoline, a carcinogen, can show up as a contaminant in disperse-dyed products. (p. 192)

Raynaud's—A condition related to autoimmune disease that involves a loss of blood flow to fingers and other extremities. (pp. 1, 43)

REACH—The European Union's Registration, Evaluation, Authorisation and Restriction of Chemicals. Enacted in 2006, it is meant to help protect the health of Europeans and the environment from the negative impacts of uncontrolled chemical use and release. European companies that import or sell chemical products or products with hazardous chemicals are compelled to identify and manage that risk, plus communicate safety measures to users. If a chemical's risks cannot be managed, it is restricted. The long-term goal is for most hazardous substances to be substituted with safer alternatives. (pp. 191, 192, 200, 222)

Regrettable substitution—When one chemical is deemed unsafe for use in consumer products, a chemical with a similar structure is substituted, until research shows it has similar health effects, and another similar chemical is substituted, and so forth . . . (pp. 78, 122)

Reprotoxic—Can cause birth defects or damage the reproductive system. (pp. 10, 121)

Restricted substance list (RSL)—A list of chemicals that are not allowed in or on a consumer product, or that are allowed only when detected by tests up to a certain limit. This limit is usually listed in ppm (parts per million) or µg/g (microgram per gram), which have a one-to-one conversion (i.e., 1 ppm = 1 µg/g). (pp. 55, 199, 213, 248)

Safety data sheet (SDS)—Formerly known as material safety data sheets (MSDSs); chemical manufacturers and sellers provide SDSs to users of their chemical products. They include the chemical product's properties, its physical and health hazards, its environmental hazards, and how to safely handle, store, and transport it. They often do not include what basic chemical components the chemical product contains, or their CAS numbers. (p. 169)

Scivera—A company that provides brands with chemistry certifications and toxicology risk screening for consumer products. (pp. 196, 199, 207)

Screened Chemistry—A service provided by Scivera and ToxServices. Chemical companies provide the chemical makeup of their products straight to Scivera or ToxServices, and these companies in turn provide a risk assessment report to brands on the potentially hazardous properties of all the chemicals used in the manufacture and finishing of those products. Brands can then request a reformulation or alternatives from chemical companies in order to bring the risk down to a level they are comfortable with.

Short-chain per- and polyfluoroalkyl substances—Possessing six instead of eight or more carbon atoms. Although short-chain PFAS were first thought to be less persistent than long-chain PFAS and thus safe for use on consumer products, emerging research shows health effects similar to long-chain PFOA and PFOS. Not yet banned at the federal level in the

United States as of October 2022. Voluntarily phased out by a handful of fashion brands. (p. 89)

Synthetic fiber—A fiber created from fossil fuel sources; examples include polyester, PVC, polyurethane, nylon, and acrylic. (pp. 76, 107, 217)

Teflon—A brand name of chemical coating, scientific name polytetrafluoroethylene (PTFE). While most famous for its use in nonstick cookware, it has also been used as a durable water and stain repellent for textiles, especially in uniforms and outdoor gear. While Chemours, a company spun off Du-Pont, has moved away from long-chain PFAS, Teflon still employs short-chain PFAS. (pp. 16, 21, 86, 88, 89)

Toluene—A volatile organic compound (VOC) that is commonly restricted for use in fashion manufacturing. Associated with solvent-based processes such as polyurethane coatings and glues. Linked to birth defects and pregnancy loss, liver damage, and central nervous system damage. (pp. 26, 103, 171, 183, 242)

Toxicant-induced loss of tolerance (TILT)—Sometimes diagnosed as multiple chemical sensitivity or mast cell activation syndrome, a condition in which overexposure to a chemical substance sensitizes the body so that being re-exposed to even a tiny amount triggers several reactions, including brain fog, hives, debilitating fatigue, and pain. (pp. 133, 137, 139, 141, 143, 153, 178, 242)

Toxic Substances Control Act (TSCA)—Legislation passed in 1976 that set up a framework for assessing and controlling toxic chemicals in the United States. Seen by many as too lax, it permitted an estimated sixty-four thousand commercially available chemicals. (pp. 87, 112, 189, 229)

Tributyl phosphate (TBP)—Also known as phosphoric acid tributyl ester or tri-n-butyl phosphate. Can cause respiratory and skin problems. Present in aviation hydraulic fluid. In fashion, used as a wetting agent and solvent. (pp. 21, 22, 26)

ZDHC—An initialism for Zero Discharge of Hazardous Chemicals, ZDHC was founded in 2011 as an industry group of a half dozen large brands dedicated to cleaning up the effluent of fashion manufacturers by specifying what chemicals are not allowed to be used in the supply chain through its MRSL and regular effluent testing. It now includes two hundred global brands, suppliers, chemical manufacturers, NGOs, trade associations, auditors, and labs. (pp. 55, 166–67, 169, 172, 184, 188, 211, 214, 226, 248)

ACKNOWLEDGMENTS

I'm so fortunate to have a team of the most kind, enthusiastic, and—above all—skilled women around me who helped usher this book into being. Whether as an editor or book agent, Georgia King has quite honestly been my career fairy godmother, kicking all this off with such a simple question: "So what will your book be about?"

Going back even further, thank you to my husband for being so invested in my happiness that he memorized the publications I wanted to write for and, when he met Georgia—then the editor at one of those publications—sent me over to pitch her before she walked out the door.

Thank you to the delightful Kate Mack, who as my agent makes me feel so well cared for. Michelle Howry, my famously wonderful book editor, has lived up to her reputation with her reassuring attitude and hands-on work wrangling my overenthusiastic reporting into something readable. Thank you to Hannah Murphy Winter, who meticulously fact-checked this book from end to end, and in the process pushed me to go even deeper to understand and communicate accurately this new and complex science; and Heather Rodino, who not only caught all my dumb spelling and grammar mistakes but left the most encouraging notes and even added to my reporting! Thank you to Sujatha Sivagnanam, my indispensable guide into the beautiful complexity of Coimbatore and Tirupur, and the several journalists who sent me to her.

Thank you to Alexandra McNair of the nonprofit Fashion FWD for opening her research notebook to me at the beginning of this process several years ago, Jasmin Malik Chua for enthusiastically pointing me in all the right directions and providing some of the best reporting on sustainable fashion news available, and Heather Poole for connecting me to several flight attendants who provided their stories for the book. Speaking of, I'm so grateful to all the people who opened up to me about their sometimes quite traumatic experiences. You'll find several of their names in this book, but there were many more who gifted me their time whom I either could not name for privacy reasons, or I could not include. No story was wasted—each added to my understanding and inspired me to work harder.

Thank you to Judith Anderson and the Association of Flight Attendants for their hard work not only supporting attendants but meticulously documenting every detail and then, on top of that, trusting me to share those details with the world.

I'm grateful to have had access to such extensive information on historical fashion toxicity and current health issues through the books of Maxine Bédat, Alison Matthews David, Dan Fagin, Simon Garfield, Eleanor Herman, Donna Jackson Nakazawa, Shanna H. Swan and Stacey Colino, and Meghan O'Rourke. I could not have made the connections I did without leaning on the impressive primary research these authors conducted.

I would like to give a shout-out to all the local journalists who have reported on toxic chemical exposures in their communities. Their reporting forms the backbone of much of this book. Please go out and subscribe to your local newspaper today; community-oriented journalism desperately needs your support.

Thank you to the current and former teammates at EcoCult, who together kept the website going while I buried myself in the work of researching and writing this thing.

I would like to thank my family, those who are still with us and those who have left us, a small unit of book-loving nerds who modeled for me the deep pleasures of devouring a good nonfiction book over breakfast, on the beach, in the car . . . anytime, really. And last but certainly not least, I would like to express my deep affection and love for my weird and wonderful friends—you know who you are. Our funny, beautiful, emotional, creative times together have kept me present, sane, and grounded in what is important.

NOTES

INTRODUCTION

4   **Today our rivers and air:** "The Clean Air Act: Successes and Challenges Since 1970," January 6, 2020, https://www.rff.org/news/press-releases/clean-air-act-successes-and-challenges-1970/.

5   **Organic food promising to be:** Samantha Oller, "Organic Food Sales Growth Slowed in 2021 as Consumer Priorities Shifted," Food Dive, June 10, 2022, https://www.fooddive.com/news/organic-food-sales-growth-slows-2021/624994/.

5   **Yet fashion, a $2.5-trillion:** Maxine Bédat, *Unraveled: The Life and Death of a Garment* (New York: Portfolio/Penguin, 2021).

6   **In 2011 (the last time industrial pollution:** Alden Wicker, "Nope, Fashion Is Not Responsible for 20% of Global Water Pollution, Either," *Ecocult* (blog), July 27, 2022, https://ecocult.com/fashion-20-percent-global-water-pollution/.

6   **In 2012, Greenpeace followed that bombshell:** Greenpeace International, *Toxic Threads: The Big Fashion Stitch-Up*, November 20, 2012, https://www.greenpeace.org/international/publication/6889/toxic-threads-the-big-fashion-stitch-up.

6   **and its #whomademyclothes campaign:** #MoveMe, "#WhoMadeMyClothes Online Social Media Movement," accessed August 24, 2022, https://moveme.berkeley.edu/project/whomademyclothes/.

10   **At least 40,000 chemicals are used commercially:** Gregory G. Bond, "How Do We Calculate the Number of Chemicals in Use Around the Globe?" International Council of Chemical Associations (ICCA) (blog), May 20, 2020, https://icca-chem.org/news/how-do-we-calculate-the-number-of-chemicals-in-use-around-the-globe/.

10   **Some researchers have warned:** Linn Persson, Bethanie M. Carney Almroth, Christopher D. Collins, Sarah Cornell, Cynthia A. de Wit, Miriam L. Diamond, Peter Fantke, et al., "Outside the Safe Operating Space of

the Planetary Boundary for Novel Entities," *Environmental Science & Technology* 53, no. 3 (January 18, 2022), https://doi.org/10.1021/acs .est.1c04158.

10 **The chemical industry is now:** IEA, "Chemicals—Fuels & Technologies," accessed August 24, 2022, https://www.iea.org/fuels-and -technologies/chemicals.

10 **petrochemicals are predicted:** IEA, "The Future of Petrochemicals— Analysis," accessed August 17, 2022, https://www.iea.org/reports/the -future-of-petrochemicals.

CHAPTER 1

18 **"It's not a new fabric,":** Steve Vogel, "New TSA Uniforms Trigger a Rash of Complaints," *Washington Post*, January 5, 2009, http://www .washingtonpost.com/wp-dyn/content/article/2009/01/05/AR2009 010502146.html.

20 **Anderson receives weekly reports:** Kathleen Doheny, "Lobbying for Fewer Bad Air Days Aloft—Los Angeles Times," *Los Angeles Times*, February 27, 2000, https://www.latimes.com/archives/la-xpm-2000-feb -27-tr-3029-story.html.

22 **Greenpeace found it:** "Dirty Laundry: Unraveling the Corporate Connections to Toxic Water Pollution in China," Greenpeace International, 2011, https://www.greenpeace.org/international/publication/7168 /dirty-laundry/.

22 **Only Levi's specifies a limit for tributyl phosphate:** Restricted Substance List, Levi Strauss & Co., January 2020.

28 **The thing is, Harvard researchers:** Eileen McNeely, Steven J. Staffa, Irina Mordukhovich, and Brent Coull, "Symptoms Related to New Flight Attendant Uniforms," *BMC Public Health* 17, no. 1 (December 2017): 972, https://doi.org/10.1186/s12889-017-4982-4.

32 **In the US, one in eight women:** Breastcancer.org, "Breast Cancer Facts and Statistics," July 14, 2022, https://www.breastcancer.org/facts -statistics.

32 **the same number will develop thyroid issues:** American Thyroid Association, "General Information/Press Room," *American Thyroid Association* (blog), accessed August 23, 2022, https://www.thyroid.org/media -main/press-room/.

32 **thyroid cancer was also:** American Thyroid Association, "World Thyroid Day Is Heralded by International Thyroid Societies," *American Thyroid Association* (blog), May 19, 2015, https://www.thyroid.org /world-thyroid-day-is-heralded-by-international-thyroid-societies/.

32 **About 70 to 90 percent of cancer cases:** Honor Whiteman, "Most Cancer Cases 'Caused by Lifestyle, Environment—Not Bad Luck,'" Medical News Today, December 17, 2015, https://www.medicalnewstoday .com/articles/304230.

32 **men are also suffering:** Miranda Bryant, "Falling Sperm Counts 'Threaten Human Survival,' Expert Warns," *Guardian*, February 26, 2021, https://www.theguardian.com/us-news/2021/feb/26/falling -sperm-counts-human-survival.

CHAPTER 2

40   **making up 70 percent:** Kirsten E. Overdahl, David Gooden, Benjamin Bobay, Gordon J. Getzinger, Heather M. Stapleton, and P. Lee Ferguson, "Characterizing Azobenzene Disperse Dyes in Commercial Mixtures and Children's Polyester Clothing," *Environmental Pollution* 287 (October 15, 2021): 117299, https://doi.org/10.1016/j.envpol.2021.117299.

41   **"In 1998, for example:** Nena Baker, *The Body Toxic: How the Hazardous Chemistry of Everyday Things Threatens Our Health and Well-Being* (New York: North Point Press, 2009), 197.

41   **the EPA almost completely stopped posting:** "EPA Re-Initiates Publication of Chemical Health and Safety Notices to ChemView, Enhancing Public Accessibility," US EPA, February 3, 2022, https://www.epa.gov/chemicals-under-tsca/epa-re-initiates-publication-chemical-health-and-safety-notices-chemview.

42   **Some azo dyes are known skin sensitizers:** Amit Bafana, Sivanesan Saravana Devi, and Tapan Chakrabarti, "Azo Dyes: Past, Present and the Future," *Environmental Reviews* 19 (2011): 350–70.

42   **First of all, some companies argue:** NimkarTek Blog, "Banned Amines in Textile and Leather," August 11, 2015, http://nimkartek.com/blog/banned-amines-in-textile-and-leather/.

44   **It's estimated that:** Gregory G. Bond, "How Do We Calculate the Number of Chemicals in Use Around the Globe?" International Council of Chemical Associations (ICCA), accessed August 24, 2022, https://icca-chem.org/news/how-do-we-calculate-the-number-of-chemicals-in-use-around-the-globe/.

47   **contact with a product as little as once a week:** Brandon L. Adler and Vincent A. DeLeo, "Allergic Contact Dermatitis," *JAMA Dermatology* 157, no. 3 (2021): 364.

49   **As the author said:** Jane E. Brody, "Solving the Mystery of I.B.S.," *New York Times,* August 2, 2021, https://www.nytimes.com/2021/08/02/well/live/irritable-bowel-syndrome-treatments-causes.html.

49   **But according to the Mayo Clinic:** "Crohn's Disease—Symptoms and Causes—Mayo Clinic," accessed August 24, 2022, https://www.mayoclinic.org/diseases-conditions/crohns-disease/symptoms-causes/syc-20353304.

49   **A new theory posits:** Brody, "Solving the Mystery of I.B.S.," https://www.nytimes.com/2021/08/02/well/live/irritable-bowel-syndrome-treatments-causes.html.

53   **and other research showed that:** Stéphanie Crettaz, Patrick Kämpfer, Beat J. Brüschweiler, Susanne Nussbaumer, and Otmar Deflorin, "Survey on Hazardous Non-Regulated Aromatic Amines as Cleavage Products of Azo Dyes Found in Clothing Textiles on the Swiss Market," *Journal of Consumer Protection and Food Safety* 15, no. 1 (March 1, 2020): 49–61, https://doi.org/10.1007/s00003-019-01245-1.

53   **The French Agency for Food, Environmental and Occupational Health & Safety:** Anses—Agence nationale de sécurité sanitaire de l'alimentation, de l'environnement et du travail, "Chemicals in Textiles and Footwear: A Proposal for Regulations That Offer More Protection,"

March 9, 2022, https://www.anses.fr/en/content/chemicals-textiles-and
-footwear-proposal-regulations-offer-more-protection.

54 **But a 2011 lawsuit alleged:** Webb v. Carter's Inc., 272 F.R.D. 489, C.D.
Cal., Judgment, Law, casemine.com, No. CV 08-7367 GAF (MaNx), accessed August 24, 2022.

55 **Carter's only gesture toward taking responsibility:** Lisa Arneill,
"CPSC and Carter's Advise Parents of Rashes Associated with Heat
Transferred, or 'Tag-Less,' Labels," *Growing Your Baby* (blog), October
24, 2008, https://www.growingyourbaby.com/cpsc-and-carter's-advise
-parents-of-rashes-associated-with-heat-transferred-or-"tag-less"-labels/.

55 **In 2019, the advocacy organization Green America:** "Green America:
Carter's Responds to Calls to Remove Toxic Chemicals from Baby
Clothes, Improve Sustainability Practices," April 9, 2020, https://www
.businesswire.com/news/home/20200409005488/en/Green-America
-Carter%E2%80%99s-Responds-to-Calls-to-Remove-Toxic-Chemicals
-From-Baby-Clothes-Improve-Sustainability-Practices.

55 **Victoria's Secret's rejoinder was:** South Florida *Sun-Sentinel*, "Victoria's
Secret," *Chicago Tribune*, April 8, 2009, https://www.chicagotribune
.com/lifestyles/health/sns-health-victorias-secret-bras-hurt-story
.html.

55 **"It would be awesome if garment manufacturers:** Debra DeAngelo,
"Victoria's Secret Responds to Rash Issue with Win-Win Suggestion,"
Davis Enterprise, July 11, 2015, https://www.davisenterprise.com/fo
rum/opinion-columns/victorias-secret-responds-to-rash-issue-with-win
-win-suggestion/.

55 **The brand might have heeded this warning:** Simon Glover, "ZDHC
Foundation Names Top Performing Brands," Ecotextile News, June 17,
2022, https://www.ecotextile.com/2022061729497/dyes-chemicals
-news/zdhc-foundation-names-top-performing-brands.html.

CHAPTER 3

62 **according to Eleanor Herman's book:** Eleanor Herman, *The Royal Art
of Poison: Filthy Palaces, Fatal Cosmetics, Deadly Medicine, and Murder
Most Foul* (New York: St. Martin's Press, 2018).

63 **The powerful Borgia family:** Marianna Karamanou, George Androut-
sos, A. Wallace Hayes, and Aristides Tsatsakis, "Toxicology in the Borgias
Period: The Mystery of Cantarella Poison," *Toxicology Research and
Application* 2 (January 1, 2018): 2397847318771126, https://doi.org
/10.1177/2397847318771126.

63 **All of them relied mainly:** Karamanou et al., "Toxicology in the Borgias
Period."

64 **The gloves were dipped in boiled animal fat:** Fracesca Scantlebury,
"Catherine de' Medici's Scented Gloves," *Costume Society* (blog), accessed
August 25, 2022, https://costumesociety.org.uk/blog/post/catherine-de
-medicis-scented-gloves.

64 **infused with jasmine, orange blossom:** Herman, *Royal Art of Poison*.

66 **In 1857, a sixty-one-year-old hatter:** Alison Matthews David, *Fashion
Victims: The Dangers of Dress Past and Present*, 3rd ed., (London: Bloomsbury Visual Arts, 2015), 60.

67 **If a few working-class men had the shakes:** Thomas Le Roux, "The Erasure of the Worker's Body: Health in the Workplace During the Early Industrialization of Paris (1770–1840)," *Le Mouvement Social* 234, no. 1 (March 22, 2011): 103–19.

68 **One workshop that Tenon visited:** Matthews David, *Fashion Victims.* Calculated from p. 56.

68 **When modern conservators:** Graham Martin and Marion Kite, "Potential for Human Exposure to Mercury and Mercury Compounds from Hat Collections," *AICCM Bulletin* 30 (December 1, 2006): 12–16, https://doi.org/10.1179/bac.2006.30.1.002.

69 **Its symptoms:** Kevin M. Rice, Ernest M. Walker, Miaozong Wu, Chris Gillette, and Eric R. Blough, "Environmental Mercury and Its Toxic Effects," *Journal of Preventive Medicine and Public Health* 47, no. 2 (March 2014): 74–83, https://doi.org/10.3961/jpmph.2014.47.2.74.

69 **To this day, there's no standard list of symptoms:** Alexandre Malek, Krystel Aouad, Rana El Khoury, Maya Halabi-Tawil, and Jacques Choucair, "Chronic Mercury Intoxication Masquerading as Systemic Disease: A Case Report and Review of the Literature," *European Journal of Case Reports in Internal Medicine* 4, no. 6 (May 24, 2017): 000632, https://doi.org/10.12890/2017_000623.

69 **In 1941, a year after *The American Public Health Report*:** Shirley T. Wajda, "Ending the Danbury Shakes: A Story of Workers' Rights and Corporate Responsibility," Connecticut History, a CTHumanities Project, December 12, 2020, https://connecticuthistory.org/ending-the-danbury-shakes-a-story-of-workers-rights-and-corporate-responsibility/.

69 **The last hat factory:** Linda Stowell, "Last Hat Factory in 'Hat City' Closes," AP News, December 18, 1987, https://apnews.com/article/a56e970a90b5d28fd928836acfd68184.

70 **I first read about Debbie:** Brianna Snyder, "Gloversville Tanneries Fade Away, but Illness Remains," *Times Union*, July 6, 2016, https://www.timesunion.com/news/article/Gloversville-tanneries-fade-away-but-illness-8343901.php.

71 **Many tanneries in Europe used:** J. G. P., "The Puering, Bating, and Drenching of Skins," *Nature* 90, no. 2240 (October 1912): 130, https://doi.org/10.1038/090130a0.

71 **Some traditional tanneries in Morocco:** AFAR, "Chouara Tannery," accessed October 18, 2022, https://www.afar.com/places/chouara-tannery.

71 **Tanners could also substitute high-tannin materials:** "Chrome Tanned vs. Vegetable Tanned Leather, Explained," Gentleman's Gazette, YouTube video, August 3, 2020, https://www.youtube.com/watch?v=6D3TrHqhJHw.

71 **Around that time, in 1853:** Jennifer Mazur, "Historic Gloversville," City of Gloversville, June 2, 2015, http://www.cityofgloversville.com/category/historic-gloversville/.

72 **The creek was devoid of life:** Snyder, "Gloversville Tanneries Fade Away," https://www.timesunion.com/news/article/Gloversville-tanneries-fade-away-but-illness-8343901.php."

72 **"They said our city smelled so bad:** Debbie M. Price, "In Upstate New York, Life Under Leather's Long Shadow," *Undark Magazine*, February

22, 2017, https://undark.org/2017/02/22/leathers-long-shadow-gloversville-new-york/.

72 **When Debbie was in middle school:** Debbie M. Price, "Our Lust for Leather Comes at a High Price in the Developing World," *Undark Magazine*, February 21, 2017, https://undark.org/2017/02/21/leather-tanning-bangladesh-india/.

74 **Chronic chromium VI poisoning:** "Chromium (Cr) Toxicity: Clinical Assessment—History, Signs and Symptoms," ATSDR, February 9, 2021, https://www.atsdr.cdc.gov/csem/chromium/signs_and_symptoms.html.

76 **One of its first uses was for mustard gas–resistant garments:** "Introduction to Polyurethanes: History," American Chemistry Council, accessed July 28, 2021, https://polyurethane.americanchemistry.com/History/.

76 **In 1926, Waldo Lonsbury Semon:** Mary Bellis, "Explore the History and Evolution of Vinyl," *ThoughtCo* (blog), February 19, 2019, https://www.thoughtco.com/history-of-vinyl-1992458.

76 **By 1959, industry scientists were concerned:** Jennifer Beth Sass, Barry Castleman, and David Wallinga, "Vinyl Chloride: A Case Study of Data Suppression and Misrepresentation," *Environmental Health Perspectives* 113, no. 7 (July 2005): 809–12, https://doi.org/10.1289/ehp.7716.

77 **British designer Mary Quant:** "Six Revolutionary Designs by Mary Quant," Victoria and Albert Museum, accessed August 25, 2022, https://www.vam.ac.uk/articles/six-revolutionary-designs-by-mary-quant.

77 **The mod designer said she was "bewitched":** "Fashion Unpicked: The 'Wet Collection' by Mary Quant," Victoria and Albert Museum, accessed August 25, 2022, https://www.vam.ac.uk/articles/fashion-unpicked-the-wet-collection-by-mary-quant.

77 **and on celebrities like Cynthia Lennon:** Kettj Talon, "The PVC Revolution in the Fashion World," *Nss Magazine* (blog), November 29, 2018, https://www.nssmag.com/en/article/16936.

77 **By the mid-1970s:** Sass, "Vinyl Chloride: A Case Study of Data Suppression and Misrepresentation."

77 **In fact, part of that seductive "new car smell":** William H. Hedley, Joseph T. Cheng, Robert J. McCormick, and Woodrow A. Lewis, "Sampling of Automobile Interiors for Vinyl Chloride Monomer," EPA, May 1976.

77 **The industry responded by secretly funding:** Sass et al., "Vinyl Chloride," https://doi.org/10.1289/ehp.7716."

78 **In the 2010s, another issue hit the headlines:** Amy Westervelt, "Phthalates Are Everywhere, and the Health Risks Are Worrying. How Bad Are They Really?," *Guardian*, February 10, 2015, https://www.theguardian.com/lifeandstyle/2015/feb/10/phthalates-plastics-chemicals-research-analysis.

78 **The "regrettable substitution" shuffle started:** Carl-Gustaf Bornehag, Fredrik Carlstedt, Bo AG J Jönsson, Christian H. Lindh, Tina K. Jensen, Anna Bodin, Carin Jonsson, Staffan Janson, and Shanna H. Swan, "Prenatal Phthalate Exposures and Anogenital Distance in Swedish Boys," *Environmental Health Perspectives* 123, no. 1 (January 2015): 101–7, https://doi.org/10.1289/ehp.1408163.

78 **But advocacy groups are still finding phthalates:** Forever Barbie Children's Clutch with Di-isodecyl phthalate (DIDP) on 07/28/2022 and children's shoes with Di(2-ethylhexyl)phthalate (DEHP) on 05/03/2022, State of California Department of Justice, Office of the Attorney General, "Proposition 65 60-Day Notice Search Results," accessed August 25, 2022, https://oag.ca.gov/prop65/60-day-notice-search-results.

79 **Ruth Benerito was born Ruth Rogan:** "Ruth Benerito," Science History Institute, December 1, 2017, https://www.sciencehistory.org/historical-profile/ruth-benerito.

80 **Benerito's team was put on the task:** Lauren K. Wolf, "What's That Stuff? Wrinkle-Free Cotton," *Chemical & Engineering News*, December 2, 2013, https://cen.acs.org/articles/91/i48/Wrinkle-Free-Cotton.html.

80 **And using her method:** "Ruth R. Benerito, 2002 Lemelson-MIT Lifetime Achievement Award Winner," Lemelson Foundation, YouTube video, March 1, 2009, https://www.youtube.com/watch?v=wOUZZu7CoTI.

80 **Polyester ended up taking the lion's share:** Michael Sadowski, Lewis Perkins, and Emily McGarvey, "Roadmap to Net Zero: Delivering Science-Based Targets in the Apparel Sector," World Resources Institute, November 2021, https://www.wri.org/research/roadmap-net-zero-delivering-science-based-targets-apparel-sector.

81 **We can smell it:** Amanda Grennell, "Does Formaldehyde Cause Leukemia? A Delayed EPA Report May Hold the Answer," *NewsHour*, PBS, August 29, 2018, https://www.pbs.org/newshour/science/does-formaldehyde-cause-leukemia-a-delayed-epa-report-may-hold-the-answer.

81 **In 1981, Americans saw a minute-long TV commercial:** "Visa Fabrics Commercial, 1980's," YouTube video, October 28, 2014, https://www.youtube.com/watch?v=tYxxCbtfzHY.

82 **according to a Forbes estimate:** Alyssa A. Lappen, "Can Roger Milliken Emulate William Randolph Hearst?," *Forbes*, May 29, 1989, http://www.alyssaalappen.org/1989/05/29/can-roger-milliken-emulate-william-randolph-hearst/.

82 **In the 1960s, roughly 95 percent:** Stephanie Clifford, "U.S. Textile Plants Return, with Floors Largely Empty of People," *New York Times*, September 19, 2013, https://www.nytimes.com/2013/09/20/business/us-textile-factories-return.html.

83 **A 2012 report from the German Federal Institute for Risk Assessment:** "Introduction to the Problems Surrounding Garment Textiles," Bundesinstitut für Risikobewertung, July 6, 2012, https://www.bfr.bund.de/cm/349/introduction-to-the-problems-surrounding-garment-textiles.pdf.

84 **In the 1980s, a study of people:** Grennell, "Does Formaldehyde Cause Leukemia?" https://www.pbs.org/newshour/science/does-formaldehyde-cause-leukemia-a-delayed-epa-report-may-hold-the-answer.

84 **The Government Accountability Office:** Tara Siegel Bernard, "When Wrinkle-Free Clothing Also Means Formaldehyde Fumes," *New York Times*, December 11, 2010, https://www.nytimes.com/2010/12/11/your-money/11wrinkle.html.

85   **Though, ever on top of trends:** "Breathe by Milliken," Milliken, accessed August 1, 2020, https://www.millikenspecialtyinteriors.com /breathe-by-milliken/.

85   **In 2018, tensions flared again when the EPA:** Grennell, "Does Formaldehyde Cause Leukemia?" https://www.pbs.org/newshour/science /does-formaldehyde-cause-leukemia-a-delayed-epa-report-may-hold-the -answer.

85   **In 2014, Milliken bought an old textile plant in Georgia:** "Flame Resistant Fabric, FR Fabric Brands, Westex: A Milliken Brand," accessed August 8, 2021, https://www.westex.com/fr-fabric-brands/?gclid=CjwK CAjwgb6IBhAREiwAgMYKRjlHdXbCZXGHkhicl7lDJol5k0ElJ9U9X cAPzGtqEh_bNskFqhKFSxoCQ8wQAvD_BwE.

85   **In 2011, the worst fish kill in Georgia's history:** Jim Abbot, "The Fishkill on Georgia's Ogeechee River," Scalawag, May 24, 2018, http:// scalawagmagazine.org/2018/05/the-fishkill-on-georgias-ogeechee -river/.

85   **Even after Milliken revamped:** Laura Corley, "Milliken Asks to Lower Pollution Permit Standards for Ogeechee River Plant," *The Current*, October 28, 2020, http://thecurrentga.org/2020/10/28/milliken-asks -to-lower-pollution-permit-standards-for-ogeechee-river-plant/.

85   **on its glossy corporate sustainability website:** "Milliken Sustainability," Milliken, accessed August 8, 2021, https://sustainability.milliken.com/.

86   **So in September 2020, Milliken put in a request:** Corley, "Milliken Asks to Lower Pollution Permit Standards for Ogeechee River Plant."

86   **This astounded the Ogeechee community:** Georgia Department of Natural Resources Environmental Protection Division, Public Hearing Proposed NPDES Permit, King America Finishing, Inc., 2020.

86   **The American chemical company 3M invented:** Nathaniel Rich, "The Lawyer Who Became DuPont's Worst Nightmare," *New York Times Magazine*, January 6, 2016, https://www.nytimes.com/2016/01/10 /magazine/the-lawyer-who-became-duponts-worst-nightmare.html.

88   **PFOA has been found in animals in the Antarctic:** Sharon Lerner, "The Teflon Toxin: DuPont and the Chemistry of Deception," *The Intercept*, August 11, 2015, https://theintercept.com/2015/08/11/dupont -chemistry-deception/.

88   **It's in the rainwater:** Matt McGrath, "Pollution: 'Forever Chemicals' in Rainwater Exceed Safe Levels," BBC News, August 2, 2022m, https:// www.bbc.com/news/science-environment-62391069.

88   **Paul Cotter, a firefighter from Massachusetts:** Hiroko Tabuchi, "Firefighters Battle an Unseen Hazard: Their Gear Could Be Toxic," *New York Times*, January 26, 2021, https://www.nytimes.com/2021/01/26/cli mate/pfas-firefighter-safety.html.

89   **In an email to a Nantucket firefighter:** Ariel Wittenberg, "Firefighters Face Lies, 'Phony' Studies on PFAS Exposure," *E&E News*, February 17, 2021, https://subscriber.politicopro.com/article/eenews/1063725299.

90   **first in a Sierra Club investigation:** Jessian Choy, "What You Need to Know About 'Nontoxic' Menstrual Underwear," *Sierra* magazine, March 16, 2020, https://www.sierraclub.org/sierra/what-you-need -know-about-nontoxic-menstrual-underwear.

92 **That led to an industry-rocking 2017 study:** Laurel A. Schaider, Simona A. Balan, Arlene Blum, David Q. Andrews, Mark J. Strynar, Margaret E. Dickinson, David M. Lunderberg, Johnsie R. Lang, and Graham F. Peaslee, "Fluorinated Compounds in U.S. Fast Food Packaging," *Environmental Science & Technology Letters* 4, no. 3 (2017): 105–11, https://doi.org/10.1021/acs.estlett.6b00435.

93 **It announced that it would phase out:** Betsy Sikma, "Milliken & Company Commits to Eliminating PFAS," Milliken, accessed August 25, 2022, https://www.milliken.com/en-us/businesses/textile/news/milliken-and-company-commits-to-eliminating-pfas.

CHAPTER 4

94 **On a November morning:** Alison Matthews David, *Fashion Victims: The Dangers of Dress Past and Present*, 3rd ed., (London: Bloomsbury Visual Arts, 2020).

95 **Her condition:** Arthur Hill Hassall, "On the Danger of Green Paint in Artificial Leaves and Flowers," *American Journal of the Medical Sciences* 41, no. 81 (January 1861): 290–91, https://doi.org/10.1097/00000441-186101000-00096.

95 **Matilda had fallen ill four times:** Matthews David, *Fashion Victims.*

95 **As one of her compatriots sobbed:** "*English Woman's Journal* (1858–1864), July 1861, Edition 1 of 1, Page 314," Nineteenth-Century Serials Edition, accessed July 8, 2021, https://ncse.ac.uk/periodicals/ewj/issues/ewj_01071861/page/26/.

95 **As Romanticism, which emphasized:** Matthews David, *Fashion Victims.*

96 **While the public was well aware:** José Ramón Bertomeu Sánchez, "Chapter 5, Arsenic in France. The Cultures of Poison During the First Half of the Nineteenth Century," University of Valencia, 2018, https://www.researchgate.net/publication/345017583_5_Arsenic_in_France_The_Cultures_of_Poison_During_the_First_Half_of_the_Nineteenth_Century.

96 **It took an "accidental" death:** Matthews David, *Fashion Victims.*

97 **Some ladies of the late 1800s:** Hassall, "On the Danger of Green Paint in Artificial Leaves and Flowers," https://doi.org/10.1097/00000441-186101000-00096.

97 **In June 1862:** Matthews David, *Fashion Victims*, 72.

98 **"The colouring matter:** J. & A. Churchill, "Arsenical Ball Wreaths," *Medical Times and Gazette* 1 (1862): 139.

98 **After a teenager died:** Matthews David, *Fashion Victims*, 72.

98 **In fact, arsenic could be found:** Dan Fagin, *Toms River: A Story of Science and Salvation* (New York: Island Press, 2015).

99 **In 1870, concerned about reports:** Simon Garfield, *Mauve: How One Man Invented a Colour That Changed the World* (London: Faber and Faber, 2000), 100.

99 **It was a new field:** "Development of Physical Chemistry During the Nineteenth Century," Encyclopedia.com, accessed August 26, 2022, https://www.encyclopedia.com/science/encyclopedias-almanacs-transcripts-and-maps/development-physical-chemistry-during-nineteenth-century.

100 **An English scientist discovered:** Fagin, *Toms River*.

100 **Benzene can cause leukemia:** "Facts About Benzene," CDC, May 15, 2019, https://emergency.cdc.gov/agent/benzene/basics/facts.asp.

100 **Acute aniline poisoning:** Matthews David, *Fashion Victims*.

100 **These chemists had been working:** Fagin, *Toms River*.

100 **So the founding director of England's Royal College of Chemistry:** Fagin, *Toms River*, 115.

100 **Hofmann wanted to figure out:** Fagin, *Toms River*.

101 **fashion's palette was rather dull:** Virginia Postrel, *The Fabric of Civilization: How Textiles Made the World* (New York: Basic Books, 2020).

101 **As Simon Garfield explained in *Mauve*:** Garfield, *Mauve*.

102 **Luckily, that was the exact color:** Garfield, *Mauve*.

103 **Magazines aimed at middle-class women:** Charlotte Crosby Nicklas, "Splendid Hues: Colour, Dyes, Everyday Science, and Women's Fashion, 1840–1875," doctoral thesis, University of Brighton, 2009, https://cris.brighton.ac.uk/ws/portalfiles/portal/318269/C+Nicklas+Thesis+Final.pdf.

103 **Bloody and violent colonization:** D. P. Steensma, "'Congo' Red: Out of Africa?," *Archives of Pathology & Laboratory Medicine* 125, no. 2 (February 2001): 250–52, https://doi.org/10.5858/2001-125-0250-CR.

103 **Synthetic indigo hit the market:** Jenny Balfour-Paul, *Indigo: Egyptian Mummies to Blue Jeans* (London: Firefly Books, 2011).

103 **Later, an independent India and China:** Garfield, *Mauve*.

104 **In 1875, BASF:** Amit Bafana, Sivanesan Saravana Devi, and Tapan Chakrabarti, "Azo Dyes: Past, Present and the Future," *Environmental Reviews* 19 (2011): 350–70, https://cdnsciencepub.com/doi/abs/10.1139/a11-018.

104 **It wasn't long before reports started surfacing:** Matthews David, *Fashion Victims*, 110.

105 **But there were at least two scientists:** Garfield, *Mauve*.

106 **Thanks to Jäger and Startin:** Matthews David, *Fashion Victims*, 101.

107 **You can still see one of Jaeger's:** "Jaeger Wool Corset, 1890s," FIDM Museum, November 5, 2014, https://fidmmuseum.org/2014/11/jaeger-wool-corset-1890s.html.

107 **Starting around the mid-1800s:** Jocelyn Sears, "Wearing a 19th-Century Mourning Veil Could Result in—Twist—Death," Racked, March 29, 2018, https://www.racked.com/2018/3/29/17156818/19th-century-mourning-veil.

108 **"I have frequently been consulted:** Prince A. Morrow, A System of Genito-Urinary Diseases, Syphilology and Dermatology v. 3, 1894," https://books.google.com/books?id=s7bA2MduF5sC&pg=PR1&lpg=PR1&dq=Morrow,+%E2%80%9CA+System+of+Genito-+Urinary+Diseases,+Syphilology+and+Dermatology+v.+3,+1894,%E2%80%9D&source=bl&ots=x6LcT-gbvl&sig=ACfU3U2BexjJa7dBm9UZ25pNfOF5pRxN2w&hl=en&sa=X&ved=2ahUKEwjz6dLtnuf7AhUPK1kFHagnD_AQ6AF6BAgGEAM#v=onepage&q=Morrow%2C%20%E2%80%9CA%20System%20of%20Genito-%20Urinary%20Diseases%2C%20Syphilology%20and%20Dermatology%20v.%203%2C%201894%2C%E2%80%9D&f=false.

108 **Both the *New York Medical Journal*:** *New York Medical Journal*, vol. 50, D. Appleton & Company, 1889, https://books.google.com/books /about/New_York_Medical_Journal.html?id=FDICAAAAYAAJ.

108 **and the *Northwestern Lancet*:** *Maryland Medical Journal*, vol. 21, Harvard University 1889, https://books.google.com/books/about /Maryland_Medical_Journal.html?id=Io0RAAAAYAAJ.

108 **Between 1883 and 1894:** Sears, "Wearing a 19th-Century Mourning Veil Could Result in—Twist—Death," https://www.racked.com/2018/3 /29/17156818/19th-century-mourning-veil.

108 **And nitrobenzene:** Matthews David, *Fashion Victims*, 115.

109 **"It is essential:** Matthews David, *Fashion Victims*, 115.

110 **In the early twentieth century:** William E. Austin, *Principles and Practice of Fur Dressing and Fur Dyeing* (New York:Van Nostrand, 1922).

110 **One woman who had her eyelashes dyed:** Nena Baker, *The Body Toxic: How the Hazardous Chemistry of Everyday Things Threatens Our Health and Well-Being* (New York: North Point Press, 2009), 89.

110 **A worker died:** Matthews David, *Fashion Victims*.

110 **Dyehouse workers:** "Aniline, Medical Management Guidelines, Toxic Substance Portal," ATSDR, accessed July 15, 2021, https://wwwn.cdc .gov/TSP/MMG/MMGDetails.aspx?mmgid=448&toxid=79.

111 **In 1895, German surgeon Ludwig:** David Michaels, "Waiting for the Body Count: Corporate Decision Making and Bladder Cancer in the U.S. Dye Industry," *Medical Anthropology Quarterly* 2, no. 3 (1988): 215–32, https://doi.org/10.1525/maq.1988.2.3.02a00030.

111 **The First World War:** Garfield, *Mauve*, 110.

111 **In 1921, the International Labor Office:** Michaels, "Waiting for the Body Count," https://doi.org/10.1525/maq.1988.2.3.02a00030.

CHAPTER 5

118 **In 2020, the market for assisted reproduction:** Linu Dash and Onkar Sumant, "Assisted Reproductive Technology Market Growth by 2030," Allied Market Research, August 2021, https://www.alliedmarketresearch .com/assisted-reproductive-technology-market-A13077.

118 **Women seeking fertility treatment in the US:** Shanna H. Swan and Stacey Colino, *Count Down: How Our Modern World Is Threatening Sperm Counts, Altering Male and Female Reproductive Development, and Imperiling the Future of the Human Race* (New York: Simon & Schuster, 2020), 45.

118 **Miscarriage rates in women:** Swan and Colino, *Count Down*, 36.

118 **In the famous Wingspread Statement of 1991:** "Our Story," CHEM Trust, October 19, 2016, https://chemtrust.org/our_story/.

119 **Another study of Chinese sperm donors:** Swan and Colino, *Count Down*, 21.

119 **And they include a lot of fashion's favorite finishes and ingredients:** Saniya Rattan, Changqing Zhou, Catheryne Chiang, Sharada Mahalingam, Emily Brehm, and Jodi A. Flaws, "Exposure to Endocrine Disruptors During Adulthood: Consequences for Female Fertility," *Journal of Endocrinology* 233, no. 3 (June 2017): R109–29, https://doi.org/10.1530 /JOE-17-0023.

120 **There are more than a dozen different types of phthalates:** Rick Smith, Bruce Lourie, and Sarah Dopp, *Slow Death by Rubber Duck: The Secret Danger of Everyday Things* (Berkeley, CA: Counterpoint, 2009), 34–35.

121 **More and more researchers agree:** Barbara Demeneix, Laura N. Vandenberg, Richard Ivell, and R. Thomas Zoeller, "Thresholds and Endocrine Disruptors: An Endocrine Society Policy Perspective," *Journal of the Endocrine Society* 4, no. 10 (October 1, 2020): bvaa085, https://doi.org/10.1210/jendso/bvaa085.

121 **A July 2022 study out of Denmark:** Andreas Kortenkamp, Martin Scholze, Sibylle Ermler, Lærke Priskorn, Niels Jørgensen, Anna-Maria Andersson, and Hanne Frederiksen, "Combined Exposures to Bisphenols, Polychlorinated Dioxins, Paracetamol, and Phthalates as Drivers of Deteriorating Semen Quality," *Environment International* 165 (July 1, 2022): 107322, https://doi.org/10.1016/j.envint.2022.107322.

121 **Just reckon with the fact:** Swan and Colino, *Count Down*, 87.

121 **There's evidence that damage caused by endocrine disruptors:** Swan and Colino, *Count Down*, 139.

121 **The effect of phthalate exposure:** Swan and Colino, *Count Down*, 84.

122 **According to a 2022 study:** Jessie P. Buckley, Jordan R. Kuiper, Deborah H. Bennett, Emily S. Barrett, Tracy Bastain, Carrie V. Breton, Sridhar Chinthakindi, et al., "Exposure to Contemporary and Emerging Chemicals in Commerce Among Pregnant Women in the United States: The Environmental Influences on Child Health Outcome (ECHO) Program," *Environmental Science & Technology* 56, no. 10 (May 17, 2022): 6560–73, https://doi.org/10.1021/acs.est.1c08942.

122 **During the last few decades, one phthalate, DEHP:** Swan and Colino, *Count Down*, 125.

122 **Take DINCH:** "BASF, Hexamoll® DINCH®—the Trusted Non-Phthalate Plasticizer," BASF, YouTube video, 2016, https://www.youtube.com/watch?v=M4J5D4pMgb4.

122 **When researchers compared the number of eggs:** Swan and Colino, *Count Down*, 88.

122 **In 2021, a lab found formaldehyde:** John Mowbray, "Exclusive: Chemical Cocktail Found in Face Masks," Ecotextile News, April 1, 2021, https://www.ecotextile.com/2021040127603/dyes-chemicals-news/exclusive-chemical-cocktail-found-in-face-masks.html.

122 **In 2021, the Center for Environmental Health in California:** Arthur Friedman, "Harmful Chemical Found in 75 Sock Brands," *Sourcing Journal* (blog), November 2, 2021, https://sourcingjournal.com/topics/raw-materials/testing-california-harmful-chemical-socks-adisa-champion-reebok-new-balance-gap-310952/.

122 **In 2022, CEH tested sports bras:** Parija Kavilanz, "High Levels of Toxic Chemical Found in Sports Bras, Watchdog Warns," *CNN*, October 13, 2022, https://www.cnn.com/2022/10/13/business/bpa-sports-bras/index.html.

123 **Polyester is also at risk for containing antimony:** Jasmin Malik Chua, "'Cancer Alley' a Cautionary Tale for Fashion's Polyester Love Affair," *Sourcing Journal* (blog), July 21, 2022, https://sourcingjournal.com/sus

tainability/sustainability-news/cancer-alley-recycled-polyester-toxic
-chemicals-antimony-defend-our-health-355467/.

124 **There's evidence that conditions like polycystic ovary syndrome:** Swan
and Colino, *Count Down*, 42.

124 **2021 study out of Spain:** AFP-Relaxnews, "Some Cosmetics Could Increase the Risk of Endometriosis," FashionNetwork.com, April 7, 2021,
https://us.fashionnetwork.com/news/Some-cosmetics-could-increase
-the-risk-of-endometriosis,1293156.html.

124 **More children are being born with intersex:** Swan and Colino, *Count
Down*, 68.

124 **A study that Swan was involved in:** Swan and Colino, *Count Down*, 39.

125 **But we are exposed to them:** Swan and Colino, *Count Down*, 110.

CHAPTER 6

130 **"It was an honor to design for an iconic global aviation brand:** Ashton
Kang, "High-Flying Fashion Reaches New Heights," Delta News Hub,
May 29, 2018, https://news.delta.com/high-flying-fashion-reaches-new
-heights.

131 **"My biggest concern:** Valeriya Safronova, "Zac Posen Presents New Uniforms for Delta," *New York Times*, October 18, 2016, https://www.nytimes
.com/2016/10/20/fashion/zac-posen-delta-air-lines-new-uniforms.html.

134 **At the time of Randolph's death in 1995:** Ronald Sullivan, "Theron G.
Randolph, 89, Environmental Allergist," *New York Times*, October 5,
1995, https://www.nytimes.com/1995/10/05/us/theron-g-randolph
-89-environmental-allergist.html.

134 **Characterized by chronic fatigue:** "Gulf War Veterans' Medically Unexplained Illnesses," Public Health, US Department of Veterans Affairs,
Veterans' Health, accessed August 24, 2022, https://www.publichealth
.va.gov/exposures/gulfwar/medically-unexplained-illness.asp.

134 **this illness was present in one-third:** "Gulf War Syndrome," Johns
Hopkins Medicine, accessed August 24, 2022, https://www.hopkins
medicine.org/health/conditions-and-diseases/gulf-war-syndrome.

139 **A 1995 study of thirty-five people:** Michael K. Magill and Anthony
Suruda, "Multiple Chemical Sensitivity Syndrome," *American Family
Physician* 58, no. 3 (September 1, 1998): 721–28.

142 **the number of people diagnosed with chemical sensitivity increased:**
Anne Steinemann, "National Prevalence and Effects of Multiple Chemical
Sensitivities," *Journal of Occupational and Environmental Medicine* 60,
no. 3 (March 2018): e152–56, https://doi.org/10.1097/JOM.000000000
0001272.

142 **Miller's research team has administered:** R. F. Palmer, T. Walker, D.
Kattari, R. Rincon, R. B. Perales, C. R. Jaén, C. Grimes, D. R. Sundblad,
and C. S. Miller, "Validation of a Brief Screening Instrument for Chemical Intolerance in a Large U.S. National Sample," *International Journal
of Environmental Research and Public Health* 2021, 18, 8714, https://doi
.org/10.3390/ijerph18168714.

143 **In November of 2021, Miller:** Claudia S. Miller, Raymond F. Palmer,
Tania T. Dempsey, Nicholas A. Ashford, and Lawrence B. Afrin, "Mast
Cell Activation May Explain Many Cases of Chemical Intolerance,"

Environmental Sciences Europe 33, no. 1 (November 17, 2021): 129, https://doi.org/10.1186/s12302-021-00570-3.

CHAPTER 7

145 **The summer of 2017, Southwest Airlines debuted its kicky new uniforms:** Talia Avakian, "Southwest Just Debuted Its First New Uniforms in 20 Years," *Travel and Leisure*, June 23, 2017, https://www.travelandleisure.com/airlines-airports/southwest-airlines-new-uniforms.

147 **Tonya told a reporter:** Catherine Dunn, "'They're Hiding Something': Southwest Flight Attendant Speaks Out About Severe Reactions to Uniforms," Philly.com, March 7, 2020, https://www.inquirer.com/business/health/uniforms-toxic-rashes-southwest-american-alaska-delta-flight-attendants-20200307.html.

147 **Southwest's attendants are represented by Transport Workers:** "Local 556 History," TWU Local 556, accessed August 24, 2022, https://twu556.org/about/history/.

147 **One Southwest flight attendant:** Dunn, "'They're Hiding Something,'" https://www.inquirer.com/business/health/uniforms-toxic-rashes-southwest-american-alaska-delta-flight-attendants-20200307.html.

149 **while some of the eighty-plus autoimmune diseases:** "Autoimmune Diseases," NIH: National Institute of Allergy and Infectious Diseases, May 2, 2017, https://www.niaid.nih.gov/diseases-conditions/autoimmune-diseases.

149 **The most conservative estimate I found autoimmune disease:** "Autoimmune Disease," National Stem Cell Foundation, accessed August 24, 2022, https://nationalstemcellfoundation.org/glossary/autoimmune-disease/.

149 **Instances of children with inflammatory bowel disease and type 1 diabetes:** Committee for the Assessment of NIH Research on Autoimmune Diseases, Board on Population Health and Public Health Practice, Health and Medicine Division, and National Academies of Sciences, Engineering, and Medicine, *Enhancing NIH Research on Autoimmune Disease* (Washington, DC: National Academies Press, 2022), https://doi.org/10.17226/26554.

150 **According to the 2008 book *The Autoimmune Epidemic*:** Donna Jackson Nakazawa, *The Autoimmune Epidemic* (New York: Touchstone, 2008).

150 **According to O'Rourke's reporting:** Committee for the Assessment of NIH Research on Autoimmune Diseases, Board on Population Health and Public Health Practice, Health and Medicine Division, and National Academies of Sciences, Engineering, and Medicine, *Enhancing NIH Research on Autoimmune Disease*, https://doi.org/10.17226/26554.

151 **In 2017, 545 million people worldwide:** GBD Chronic Respiratory Disease Collaborators, "Prevalence and Attributable Health Burden of Chronic Respiratory Diseases, 1990–2017: A Systematic Analysis for the Global Burden of Disease Study 2017," *The Lancet Respiratory Medicine* 8, no. 6 (June 2020): 585–96, https://doi.org/10.1016/S2213-2600(20)30105-3.

151 **Between 1980 and 2014:** Laura Dwyer-Lindgren, Amelia Bertozzi-Villa, Rebecca W. Stubbs, Chloe Morozoff, Shreya Shirude, Mohsen Naghavi,

Ali H. Mokdad, and Christopher J. L. Murray, "Trends and Patterns of Differences in Chronic Respiratory Disease Mortality Among US Counties, 1980–2014—PMC," *Journal of the American Medical Association* 318, no. 12 (September 26, 2017): 1136–49.

151 **At least 85 percent of COPD cases:** "What Causes COPD," American Lung Association, accessed August 24, 2022, https://www.lung.org /lung-health-diseases/lung-disease-lookup/copd/what-causes-copd.

151 **researchers are linking COPD symptoms:** Nirupama Putcha, Han Woo, Meredith C. McCormack, Ashraf Fawzy, Karina Romero, Meghan F. Davis, Robert A. Wise, et al., "Home Dust Allergen Exposure Is Associated with Outcomes Among Sensitized Individuals with Chronic Obstructive Pulmonary Disease," *American Journal of Respiratory and Critical Care Medicine* 205, no. 4 (February 15, 2022): 412–20, https://doi.org /10.1164/rccm.202103-0583OC.

151 **Some doctors, according to Nakazawa's:** Nakazawa, *The Autoimmune Epidemic*, 21.

152 **Other research showed that half of women:** Nakazawa, *The Autoimmune Epidemic*, 30.

152 **Multiple studies have established:** Nakazawa, *The Autoimmune Epidemic*, 70.

152 **A cluster of multiple sclerosis cases in El Paso, Texas:** Nakazawa, *The Autoimmune Epidemic*, 117.

152 **there's evidence that endocrine disruptors:** Committee for the Assessment of NIH Research on Autoimmune Diseases, Board on Population Health and Public Health Practice, Health and Medicine Division, and National Academies of Sciences, Engineering, and Medicine, *Enhancing NIH Research on Autoimmune Disease*, https://doi.org/10.17226/26554.

CHAPTER 8

160 **It reportedly has around twenty-two thousand garment factories:** Jasmin Malik Chua, "Rising Cotton Prices Behind Indian Garment Makers' Strike Plan," *Sourcing Journal* (blog), May 5, 2022, https://sourcingjour nal.com/topics/raw-materials/india-cotton-prices-strike-tirupur-garment -owners-association-knitwear-343331/.

161 **In the late nineties, after three decades:** Adam Matthews, "The Environmental Crisis in Your Closet," *Newsweek*, August 13, 2015, https:// www.newsweek.com/2015/08/21/environmental-crisis-your-closet -362409.html.

161 **A local activist showed me:** J. Kiruthika, R. Jayasree, S. Vidhya, P. Sangeetha, and R. Sudhaa, "Comparative Study on Orathupalayam Dam Before and After Releasing of 'Contaminated' Water (Part II)," *NCSC*, Project submitted to Jaivabai Municipal Girls HR. Sec. School, Tirupur, India, 2005.

162 **The aquifer was dropping:** Neeta Deshpande, "India's Textile City of Tiruppur Is an Environmental Dark Spot," *The Wire*, February 12, 2020, https://thewire.in/environment/australian-open-tiruppur-dyeing -bleaching-groundwater-contamination-agriculture-noyyal-river.

162 **In 1996, the Supreme Court of India:** "Can the Courts Save India's Rivers from Pollution? Tirupur Shows the Answer Is No," Covai Post

Network, August 30, 2016, https://www.covaipost.com/columns/can -the-courts-save-indias-rivers-from-pollution-tirupur-shows-the -answer-is-no/.

163 **fashion trade outlets were reporting:** Chua, "Rising Cotton Prices Behind Indian Garment Makers' Strike Plan," https://sourcingjour nal.com /topics/raw-materials/india-cotton-prices-strike-tirupur-garment-owners -association-knitwear-343331/.

164 **A 2018 health survey in India:** "Hearing Loss to Tuberculosis: The Occupational Health Hazards Faced by Garment Workers," Environics Trust, accessed August 24, 2022, https://environicsindia.in/2021/07 /06/hearing-loss-to-tuberculosis-the-occupational-health-hazards -faced-by-garment-workers/.

164 **A 2021 report by researchers in Tirupur:** "Hearing Loss to Tuberculosis," Environics Trust.

164 **a type of interstitial lung disease:** David G. Kern, Eli Kern, Robert S. Crausman, and Richard W. Clapp, "A Retrospective Cohort Study of Lung Cancer Incidence in Nylon Flock Workers, 1998–2008," *International Journal of Occupational and Environmental Health* 17, no. 4 (December 2011): 345–51, https://doi.org/10.1179/107735211799 041814.

165 **In 2019, several had died:** SimpliCity News Team, "Four Youth Die of Suffocation in Tirupur: Authorities Seal Dyeing Unit," Simplicity.In, April 15, 2019, https://simplicity.in/coimbatore/english/news/46258 /Four-youth-die-of-suffocation-in-Tirupur-Authorities-seal-dyeing-unit.

165 **Garment workers who operate the machines:** Humayun Kabir, Myfanwy Maple, Kim Usher, and Md Shahidul Islam, "Health Vulnerabilities of Readymade Garment (RMG) Workers: A Systematic Review," *BMC Public Health* 19, no. 1 (January 15, 2019): 70, https://doi.org/10.1186 /s12889-019-6388-y.

165 **After Greenpeace dropped its bombshell report in 2011:** "Dirty Laundry: Unravelling the Corporate Connections to Toxic Water Pollution in China," Greenpeace International, 2011, https://www.greenpeace .org/international/publication/7168/dirty-laundry/.

166 **The next year, Greenpeace purchased:** "Toxic Threads: The Big Fashion Stitch-Up," Greenpeace International, November 20, 2012, https://www .greenpeace.org/international/publication/6889/toxic-threads-the-big -fashion-stitch-up.

166 **Almost forty of the world's largest fashion retailers:** "Contributors: Textile and Footwear Industry," Roadmap to Zero, accessed August 24, 2022, https://www.roadmaptozero.com/contributor-category/textile -and-footwear-industry.

168 **And later that year, news broke:** Simon Glover, "Mountain of Salt Sludge Hampers Dyehouses," Ecotextile News, accessed October 19, 2022, https://www.ecotextile.com/2022101029927/dyes-chemicals -news/mountain-of-salt-sludge-hampers-dyehouses.html.

169 **Earlier in 2022, a small group of organizations and companies:** Simon Glover, "H&M, Nudie in Call for Chemical Transparency," Ecotextile News, April 22, 2022, https://www.ecotextile.com/2022042229254 /dyes-chemicals-news/h-m-nudie-in-call-for-chemical-transparency.html.

172 **According to a July 2021 report by Planet Tracker:** Catherine Tubb, Nitin Sukh, and Peter Elwin, *Threadbare Data: Poor Environmental Disclosures by Textile Wet Processing Companies Prevent Investors from Properly Pricing ESG Risks and Opportunities*, Planet Tracker, May 2021, https://planet-tracker.org/environmental-data-dearth-in-wet-processing/.

172 **even the world's two hundred biggest brands:** Alden Wicker, "The Fashion Industry Could Reduce Emissions—If It Wanted To," *Wired*, November 13, 2021, https://www.wired.com/story/fashion-industry-reduce-emissions/.

173 **And these products can be contaminated:** John Mowbray, "Screening Pinpoints Textile Chemical Pollutants," Ecotextile News, November 17, 2020, https://www.ecotextile.com/2020111727003/dyes-chemicals-news/screening-pinpoints-textile-chemical-pollutants.html.

175 **In Bangladesh, where thousands of factories:** Najifa Farhat, "Hazardous Azo Dye Plagues Local Garments Market," *Dhaka Tribune*, June 4, 2022, https://www.dhakatribune.com/bangladesh/2022/06/04/hazardous-azo-dye-plagues-local-garments-market.

175 **Later, I found in a *Newsweek* article:** Matthews, "The Environmental Crisis in Your Closet," *Newsweek*, August 13, 2015. https://www.newsweek.com/2015/08/21/environmental-crisis-your-closet-362409.html.

175 **In 2016, a local newspaper:** "Can the Courts Save India's Rivers from Pollution? Tirupur Shows the Answer Is No," https://www.covaipost.com/columns/can-the-courts-save-indias-rivers-from-pollution-tirupur-shows-the-answer-is-no/.

175 **And as recently as 2020, a local researcher:** Deshpande, "India's Textile City of Tiruppur Is an Environmental Dark Spot," *The Wire*, February 12, 2020, https://thewire.in/environment/australian-open-tiruppur-dyeing-bleaching-groundwater-contamination-agriculture-noyyal-river.

176 **I told her that a similar story had played out before:** Dan Fagin, *Toms River: A Story of Science and Salvation* (New York: Island Press, 2015).

176 **That's exactly what:** FE Bureau, "Gujarat's Deep Sea Effluent Pipeline Likely to Benefit Nearly 4,500 Industrial Units," *Financial Express*, November 20, 2020, https://www.financialexpress.com/industry/gujarats-deep-sea-effluent-pipeline-likely-to-benefit-nearly-4500-industrial-units/2132449/.

CHAPTER 9

182 **Not bad, until you think about the fact:** Katie Marriner, "America's Biggest Ports Handled a Record 50.5 Million Shipping Containers Last Year," MarketWatch, February 23, 2022, https://www.marketwatch.com/story/americas-biggest-ports-handled-a-record-50-5-million-shipping-containers-last-year-11645539342.

183 **But in other countries:** Chris Baraniuk, "What Lurks Inside Shipping Containers," *Hakai Magazine*, July 7, 2022, https://hakaimagazine.com/news/what-lurks-inside-shipping-containers/.

183 **A 2017 Swedish study:** Urban Svedberg and Gunnar Johanson, "Occurrence of Fumigants and Hazardous Off-Gassing Chemicals in Shipping Containers Arriving in Sweden," *Annals of Work Exposures and Health* 61, no. 2 (March 1, 2017): 195–206, https://doi.org/10.1093/annweh /wxw022.

185 **Shein jeans:** "Incident Report Details: 20211222-CCE09-2147358340," SaferProducts.gov, December 22, 2021, https://www.saferproducts.gov /PublicSearch/Detail?ReportId=3534047.

185 **cheap jewelry:** "Incident Report Details: 20211112-93C7E-2147358801," SaferProducts.gov, November 12, 2021, https://www.saferproducts.gov /PublicSearch/Detail?ReportId=3494045.

185 **moccasins:** "Incident Report Details: 20211030-BF3E1-2147359010," SaferProducts.gov, October 30, 2021, https://www.saferproducts.gov /PublicSearch/Detail?ReportId=3484737.

185 **Skechers slip-ons:** "Incident Report Details: 20210512-13F30 -2147364164," SaferProducts.gov, May 12, 2021, https://www.saferprod ucts.gov/PublicSearch/Detail?ReportId=3281051.

185 **black $3.99 tights:** "Incident Report Details: 20201116-56398 -2147368093," SaferProducts.gov, November 16, 2021, https://www.saf erproducts.gov/PublicSearch/Detail?ReportId=2034295.

187 **Since 2016, when Congress raised the *de minimis*:** William Alan Reinsch, "De Minimis," Center for Strategic and International Studies, January 18, 2022, https://www.csis.org/analysis/de-minimis.

188 **In June 2021, a large group of surprising bedfellows:** "Joint Letter from Industry and Public Interest Groups to Congress Strongly Supporting the CPSC's Mission and a Substantial Increase in Funding," Consumer Reports Advocacy, June 2, 2021, https://advocacy.consumerreports .org/research/joint-letter-from-industry-and-public-interest-groups -to-congress-strongly-supporting-the-cpscs-mission-and-a-substantial -increase-in-funding/.

189 **The Toxic Substances Control Act of 1976:** Serena Marshall and John Parkinson, "Obama Enacts New Chemical Regulations: What Do Changes Mean?," ABC News, June 22, 2016, https://abcnews.go.com /Health/chemical-regulations/story?id=39723122.

189 **the EPA has not attempted to fully ban a chemical:** Puneet Kollipara, "The Bizarre Way the U.S. Regulates Chemicals—Letting Them on the Market First, Then Maybe Studying Them," *The Washington Post*, March 19, 2015, https://www.washingtonpost.com/news/energy-environment /wp/2015/03/19/our-broken-congresss-latest-effort-to-fix-our-broken -toxic-chemicals-law/.

189 **In 2021, whistleblowers from the EPA's New Chemicals Division:** Sharon Lerner, "EPA Division Has 'Incredibly Toxic Work Environment,'" *The Intercept*, March 30, 2022, https://theintercept.com/2022 /03/30/epa-new-chemicals-division-workplace/.

191 **The US government's approach:** Kollipara, "The Bizarre Way the U.S. Regulates Chemicals—Letting Them on the Market First, Then Maybe Studying Them," *The Washington Post*, March 19, 2015, https://www .washingtonpost.com/news/energy-environment/wp/2015/03/19 /our-broken-congresss-latest-effort-to-fix-our-broken-toxic-chemicals-law/.

191 **That's essentially what the American Apparel & Footwear Association cited:** Jasmin Malik Chua, "New York Assembly Votes to Ban PFAS From 'Common Apparel,'" *Sourcing Journal*, May 19, 2022, https://sourcingjournal.com/sustainability/sustainability-news/new-york-assembly-pfas-ban-aafa-polyfluoroalkyl-forever-chemicals-345297/.

191 **For example, it reduced industrial emissions of dioxins:** Shanna H. Swan and Stacey Colino, *Count Down: How Our Modern World Is Threatening Sperm Counts, Altering Male and Female Reproductive Development, and Imperiling the Future of the Human Race* (New York: Simon & Schuster, 2020), 199.

192 **Under Armour:** Safety Gate: the EU Rapid Alert System for Dangerous Non-food Products, "Alert Number: A12/00538/21," April 22, 2021, https://ec.europa.eu/safety-gate-alerts/screen/webReport/alertDetail/10003496.

192 **Scotch & Soda suede jacket:** Safety Gate: the EU Rapid Alert System for Dangerous Non-food Products, "Alert Number: A12/01273/20," September 24, 2020, https://ec.europa.eu/safety-gate-alerts/screen/webReport/alertDetail/10001928.

192 **In 2021, the European Chemical Agency:** Tony Whitfield, "ECHA Enforcement Finds Breaches of EU Chemical Laws," Ecotextile News, December 9, 2021, https://www.ecotextile.com/2021120828706/dyes-chemicals-news/echa-enforcement-project-finds-breaches-of-eu-chemical-laws.html.

194 **When Amazon was sued under Prop 65:** "Will Regulators Target Amazon for Prop. 65 Claims Without Section 230 Protection?," *The Recorder*, March 16, 2022, https://www.law.com/therecorder/2022/03/16/will-regulators-target-amazon-for-prop-65-claims-without-section-230-protection/?slreturn=20220724162024.

198 **There are, after all, more than twelve thousand types of PFAS:** "National PFAS Datasets," ECHO, US EPA, accessed August 24, 2022, https://echo.epa.gov/tools/data-downloads/national-pfas-datasets.

199 **And Oeko-Tex looks for:** Based on the number of perfluorochemicals in Oeko-Tex's Restricted Substance List: ECO PASSPORT by OEKO-TEX®, Edition 01.2022.

202 **But before I could make it to FedEx:** Deborah Belgum, "Counterfeits Crammed with Toxic Chemicals, AAFA Says," *Sourcing Journal* (blog), March 23, 2022, https://sourcingjournal.com/topics/compliance/toxic-chemicals-counterfeit-footwear-apparel-aafa-arsenic-lead-phthalates-cadmium-335544/.

203 **pentylphenol:** "SIN List," ChemSec, accessed August 24, 2022, https://sinlist.chemsec.org/.

205 **Just a week after I got my results:** Tom Perkins, "'Forever Chemicals' Found in Nearly 60% of Children's 'Waterproof' or 'Stain-Resistant' Textiles," *Guardian*, May 7, 2022, https://www.theguardian.com/environment/2022/may/07/pfas-forever-chemicals-children-textiles.

205 **Later that year in the fall:** Chunjie Xia, Miriam L. Diamond, Graham F. Peaslee, Hui Peng, Arlene Blum, Zhanyun Wang, Anna Shalin, et al., "Per- and Polyfluoroalkyl Substances in North American School

Uniforms," *Environmental Science & Technology* 56, no. 19 (October 4, 2022): 13845–57, https://doi.org/10.1021/acs.est.2c02111.

CHAPTER 10

212 **In September of 2022, for example, a brand called Kolan:** Jessica Binns, "Kids' Shoes Sold on Amazon Recalled for Lead Contamination," *Sourcing Journal*, September 7, 2022, https://sourcingjournal.com/foot wear/footwear-business/amazon-kolan-childrens-shoe-recall-lead-toxic -consumer-product-safety-commission-370067/.

213 **Out of the 250 largest fashion brands in the world:** "Fashion Transparency Index 2022," Fashion Revolution, August 1, 2022, https://www .fashionrevolution.org/about/transparency/.

216 **The research is still emerging:** Li-ping Wang and Jin-ye Wang, Skin Penetration of Inorganic and Metallic Nanoparticles, *Journal of Shanghai Jiaotong University (Science)* 19 (2014): 691-97, doi: 10.1007/s12204-014 -1567-6.
R. George, S. Merten, T. T. Wang, P. Kennedy, and P. Maitz, "In Vivo Analysis of Dermal and Systemic Absorption of Silver Nanoparticles Through Healthy Human Skin," *Australasian Journal of Dermatology* 55, no. 3 (2014): 185-90. doi: 10.1111/ajd.12101.

216 **A study on oral exposure:** Zannatul Ferdous and Abderrahim Nemmar, "Health Impact of Silver Nanoparticles: A Review of the Biodistribution and Toxicity Following Various Routes of Exposure," *International Journal of Molecular Sciences* 21, no. 7 (March 30, 2020): 2375, https:// doi.org/10.3390/ijms21072375.

216 **Oh, and avoid permethrin-impregnated fashion products:** Consumer Report, "How to Use Permethrin on Clothing, Safely," accessed October 6, 2022, https://www.consumerreports.org/insect-repellent/how -to-use-permethrin-on-clothing-safely-a4370607226/.

218 **A 2008 study from the University of Washington:** "Toxic Chemicals Found in Common Scented Laundry Products, Air Fresheners," Science-Daily, July 24, 2008, https://www.sciencedaily.com/releases/2008/07 /080723134438.htm.

218 **For her next 2011 study:** Anne C. Steinemann, Ian C. MacGregor, Sydney M. Gordon, Lisa G. Gallagher, Amy L. Davis, Daniel S. Ribeiro, and Lance A. Wallace, "Fragranced Consumer Products: Chemicals Emitted, Ingredients Unlisted," *Environmental Impact Assessment Review* 31, no. 3 (April 1, 2011): 328–33, https://doi.org/10.1016/j.eiar.2010.08.002.

218 **A 2002 study:** J. D. Johansen, L. Skov, A. Volund, K. Andersen, and T. Menné, "Allergens in Combination Have a Synergistic Effect on the Elicitation Response: A Study of Fragrance-Sensitized Individuals," *British Journal of Dermatology* 139, no. 2 (1998): 264–70, https://doi.org /10.1046/j.1365-2133.1998.02363.x.

219 **PERC has been shown to:** "Fact Sheet: Tetrachloroethene (PERC) in Indoor & Outdoor Air," New York State Department of Health, September 2013, https://www.health.ny.gov/environmental/chemicals /tetrachloroethene/.

221 **between 40,000 and 350,000:** Gregory G. Bond, "How Do We Calculate the Number of Chemicals in Use Around the Globe?," International

Council of Chemical Associations (ICCA), accessed August 24, 2022, https:// icca-chem.org/news/how-do-we-calculate-the-number -of-chemicals-in-use-around-the-globe/.

221   **For an example of what this could achieve:** Jim Tankersley, "A Winter-Coat Heavyweight Gives Trump's Trade War the Cold Shoulder," *New York Times*, November 23, 2018, https://www.nytimes.com/2018/11 /23/business/economy/columbia-sportswear-trump-trade-war.html.

222   **Brands like Shein:** Arthur Friedman, "Proposed de Minimis Bill 'Would Shut Down Shein,' Trade Expert Says," *Sourcing Journal*, January 19, 2022, https://sourcingjournal.com/topics/trade/de-minimis-tariff -ecommerce-china-shein-earl-blumenauer-trade-subcommittee-bill -323561/.

225   **That includes lead:** Saniya Rattan, Changqing Zhou, Catheryne Chiang, Sharada Mahalingam, Emily Brehm, and Jodi A. Flaws, "Exposure to Endocrine Disruptors During Adulthood: Consequences for Female Fertility," *Journal of Endocrinology* 233, no. 3 (June 2017): R109–29, https://doi.org/10.1530/JOE-17-0023.

226   **But when his advocacy organization:** "WA—New Study Finds Toxic Chemicals in Most Products Labeled Stain- or Water-Resistant," Toxic-Free Future, January 26, 2022, https://toxicfreefuture.org/press-room /wa-new-study-finds-toxic-chemicals-in-most-products-labeled -stain-or-water-resistant/.

CONCLUSION

232   **Eventually, 164 attendants joined the suit:** "Court Rules in Favor of Twin Hill," Twin Hill, October 3, 2016, https://www.prnewswire.com /news-releases/court-rules-in-favor-of-twin-hill-300337694.html.

233   **On October 3, 2016, Twin Hill announced:** "Court Rules in Favor of Twin Hill."

234   **In May 2017, in a town hall meeting:** Lewis Lazare, "An American Airlines Pilot Drops Bombshell About Twin Hill Uniforms," *Chicago Business Journal*, May 16, 2017, https://www.bizjournals.com/chicago /news/2017/05/16/an-american-airlines-pilot-drops-bombshell-about .html.

234   **According to Stewart Weltman:** Dan Churney, "Judge Trims, but Refuses to Ground Suit Alleging American Airlines' Uniforms Made Workers Sick," *Cook County Record*, April 28, 2020, https://cookcountyrecord .com/stories/533248071-judge-trims-but-refuses-to-ground-suit -alleging-american-airlines-uniforms-made-workers-sick.

234   **A trickle of complaints:** Zurbriggen v. Twin Hill American Airlines—Second Amended Complaint—Public (PDF), accessed August 24, 2022, https://www.scribd.com/document/395986448/Zurbriggen-v-Twin -Hill-American-Airlines-Second-Amended-Complaint-Public.

235   **So Anderson requested tests:** Association of Flight Attendants-CWA, "Uniforms," accessed October 8, 2022, https://www.afacwa.org/uni forms.

235   **By May, one out of five American Airlines attendants:** Lewis Lazare, "American Airlines' Evolving Uniform Crisis Takes Two More Surprising Turns," *Chicago Business Journal*, May 9, 2017, https://www.bizjournals

.com/chicago/news/2017/05/09/american-airlines-evolving-uniform
-crisis-takes.html.

236 **In January 2018, three years after it collected its survey data:** Eileen
McNeely, Steven J. Staffa, Irina Mordukhovich, and Brent Coull, "Symptoms Related to New Flight Attendant Uniforms," *BMC Public Health* 17,
no. 1 (December 2017): 972, https://doi.org/10.1186/s12889-017-4982-4.

237 **When, in May 2020:** "Delta Flight Attendant Uniforms Found to Contain Toxic Chemicals in Levels 10x Higher Than What's Permitted by
H&M," Paddle Your Own Kanoo, May 22, 2020, https://www.paddley
ourownkanoo.com/2020/05/22/delta-flight-attendant-uniforms
-found-to-contain-toxic-chemicals-in-levels-10x-higher-than-whats
-permitted-by-hm/.

240 **It came out in late 2020 that Girardi:** Hillel Aron, "Barely Legal: The
Surreal Saga of Tom Girardi and Erika Jayne," *Los Angeles Magazine*, November 29, 2021, https://www.lamag.com/culturefiles/the-surreal
-saga-of-tom-girardi-and-erika-jayne/.

240 **Tonya's name is spelled wrong:** On March 4, 2021, Bearup filed a "Personal Injury—Other Product Liability" lawsuit against Cintas Corporation. This case was filed in US District Courts, Ohio Southern District.
The judge overseeing this case is Matthew W. McFarland. The case status
is "Pending—Other Pending," https://unicourt.com/case/pc-db5
-bearup-v-cintas-corporation-839622.

247 **My answer is, unfortunately, you can't:** "Nobody Really Knows What
Happens to PFAS When We Throw Our Old Products Away," ChemSec,
May 12, 2022, https://chemsec.org/nobody-really-knows-what
-happens-to-pfas-when-we-throw-our-old-products-away/.

248 **Scientists have found a way to break down PFAS:** Shira Joudan and
Rylan J. Lundgren, "Taking the 'F' out of Forever Chemicals," *Science*
377, no. 6608 (August 19, 2022): 816–17, https://doi.org/10.1126/sci
ence.add1813.

248 **In August 2022, the EPA:** US EPA, OA, "EPA Proposes Designating
Certain PFAS Chemicals as Hazardous Substances Under Superfund to
Protect People's Health," news release, August 26, 2022, https://www
.epa.gov/newsreleases/epa-proposes-designating-certain-pfas-chemicals
-hazardous-substances-under-superfund.

248 **ZDHC announced in September:** Arthur Friedman, "ZDHC Adding
PFAS Chemicals to Naughty List," *Sourcing Journal* (blog), September
16, 2022, https://sourcingjournal.com/topics/raw-materials/zdhc-pfas
-chemicals-manufacturing-restricted-substances-list-textiles-footwear
-373208/.

248 **And in October:** Bay City News, "California Bans 'Forever Chemicals'
in Fabrics, Makeup," NBC Bay Area, October 2, 2022, https://www
.nbcbayarea.com/news/california/california-bans-chemicals-makeup
-fabrics/3019162/.

248 **in placentas:** Antonio Ragusa, Alessandro Svelato, Criselda Santacroce,
Piera Catalano, Valentina Notarstefano, Oliana Carnevali, Fabrizio Papa,
et al., "Plasticenta: First Evidence of Microplastics in Human Placenta,"
Environment International 146 (January 1, 2021): 106274, https://doi
.org/10.1016/j.envint.2020.106274.

248   **in human blood:** Mike Snider, "Microplastics Have Been Found in Air, Water, Food and Now . . . Human Blood," *USA Today*, March 25, 2022, https://www.usatoday.com/story/news/health/2022/03/25/plastics -found-inside-human-blood/7153385001/.

248   **in our lungs:** Damian Carrington, "Microplastics Found Deep in Lungs of Living People for First Time," *Guardian*, April 6, 2022, https://www .theguardian.com/environment/2022/apr/06/microplastics-found -deep-in-lungs-of-living-people-for-first-time.

248   **a 2022 study found that people who have inflammatory bowel disease:** Zehua Yan, Yafei Liu, Ting Zhang, Faming Zhang, Hongqiang Ren, and Yan Zhang, "Analysis of Microplastics in Human Feces Reveals a Correlation Between Fecal Microplastics and Inflammatory Bowel Disease Status," *Environmental Science & Technology* 56, no. 1 (January 4, 2022): 414–21, https://doi.org/10.1021/acs.est.1c03924.

248   **In Cambodia, according to a 2022 investigation:** "Fashion Waste from Nike, Clarks and Other Top Brands' Suppliers Burnt in Toxic Kilns Employing Modern-Day Slaves in Cambodia," Greenpeace UK, August 8, 2022, https://www.greenpeace.org.uk/news/fashion-waste -from-nike-clarks-and-other-top-brands-suppliers-burnt-in-toxic-kilns -employing-modern-day-slaves-in-cambodia/.

249   **In conscious fashion campaigner Maxine Bédat's 2021 book:** Maxine Bédat, *Unraveled: The Life and Death of a Garment* (New York: Port-folio/Penguin, 2021).

249   **Well, according to Bédat's research:** Bédat, *Unraveled*, 180.

249   **But data from the Salvation Army is even bleaker:** Bédat, *Unraveled*, 213.

249   **An estimated fifteen million items flow:** Bédat, *Unraveled*, 202.